PHOTOBIOLOGY OF INFANT SKIN

DERMATOLOGY - LABORATORY AND CLINICAL RESEARCH

Additional books in this series can be found on Nova's website at:

https://www.novapublishers.com/catalog/index.php?cPath=23_29&seriesp=
Dermatology+-+Laboratory+and+Clinical+Research

Additional e-books in this series can be found on Nova's website at:

https://www.novapublishers.com/catalog/index.php?cPath=23_29&seriespe=
Dermatology+-+Laboratory+and+Clinical+Research

DERMATOLOGY - LABORATORY AND CLINICAL RESEARCH

PHOTOBIOLOGY OF INFANT SKIN

GEORGIOS N. STAMATAS, M. CATHERINE MACK

AND

KATHARINE M. MARTIN

Nova Biomedical Press, Inc.
New York

For permission to use material from this book please contact us:
Telephone 631-231-7269; Fax 631-231-8175
Web Site: http://www.novapublishers.com

NOTICE TO THE READER
The Publisher has taken reasonable care in the preparation of this book, but makes no expressed or implied warranty of any kind and assumes no responsibility for any errors or omissions. No liability is assumed for incidental or consequential damages in connection with or arising out of information contained in this book. The Publisher shall not be liable for any special, consequential, or exemplary damages resulting, in whole or in part, from the readers' use of, or reliance upon, this material.

Independent verification should be sought for any data, advice or recommendations contained in this book. In addition, no responsibility is assumed by the publisher for any injury and/or damage to persons or property arising from any methods, products, instructions, ideas or otherwise contained in this publication.

This publication is designed to provide accurate and authoritative information with regard to the subject matter covered herein. It is sold with the clear understanding that the Publisher is not engaged in rendering legal or any other professional services. If legal or any other expert assistance is required, the services of a competent person should be sought. FROM A DECLARATION OF PARTICIPANTS JOINTLY ADOPTED BY A COMMITTEE OF THE AMERICAN BAR ASSOCIATION AND A COMMITTEE OF PUBLISHERS.

LIBRARY OF CONGRESS CATALOGING-IN-PUBLICATION DATA
Stamatas, Georgios N.
 Photobiology of infant skin / Georgios N. Stamatas, M. Catherine Mack, and
Katharine M. Martin.
      p. ; cm.
 Includes bibliographical references and index.
 ISBN 978-1-61668-751-9 (softcover)
 1. Pediatric dermatology. 2. Skin--Effect of radiation on. 3.
Infants--Health and hygiene. 4. Jaundice, Neonatal--Phototherapy. 5.
Ultraviolet radiation--Physiological effect. I. Mack, M. Catherine (Mary
Catherine) II. Martin, Katharine M. III. Title.
 [DNLM: 1. Infant. 2. Skin--radiation effects. 3. Light--adverse
effects. 4. Skin Diseases--etiology. 5. Sunlight--adverse effects. WR 102
S783p 2010]
 RJ511.S73 2010
 618.92'5--dc22
                                2010013755

Published by Nova Science Publishers, Inc. ✦ New York

CONTENTS

Preface   vii

Abbreviations   1

Chapter 1   Introduction   3

Chapter 2   Risks Associated with Exposure of Skin
             to UVR Early in Life   7

Chapter 3   Effects of UVR on the Biology of Infant Skin   13

Chapter 4   Blue Light Phototherapy for Jaundice   25

Chapter 5   Conclusion and Areas for Future Research   29

References   31

Index   49

PREFACE

The last decades have witnessed great strides in understanding the biological effects of light from the molecular all the way up to the whole organism level. Much of the boost for advancing the science of photobiology came from the dramatic increase over this period in the incidence of melanoma and other sun-related skin diseases, as well as the realization that light plays an important role in skin aging. Due to the fact that many of these conditions occur late in life, little attention has been paid to the effects of light on infant skin, with the exception of the use of violet-blue light for the treatment of jaundice in newborns. However, mounting evidence shows that a history of early sun exposure may affect the development of sun-related conditions later in life. In this chapter we summarize current knowledge about the risks of ultraviolet radiation (UVR) on infant skin, including epidemiologic evidence regarding sun exposure in this age group. Based on published results of studies performed using cell culture models, animal models, and human clinical trials, we specifically examine the effects of UVR on the biology of infant skin, as well as the known effects of blue-light phototherapy on neonatal skin. Finally, we identify areas for future research in this exciting field of science.

ABBREVIATIONS

American Academy of Pediatrics (AAP),
basal cell carcinoma (BCC),
cutaneous malignant melanoma (CMM),
deoxyribonucleic acid (DNA),
Langerhans cells (LC),
melanocytic nevi (MN),
natural moisturizing factor (NMF),
skin immune system (SIS),
solar simulated radiation (SSR),
squamous cell carcinoma (SCC),
stratum corneum (SC),
trans-epidermal water loss (TEWL),
ultraviolet radiation (UVR)

Chapter 1

INTRODUCTION

Light interacts with tissue in a plurality of ways including such phenomena as absorption, elastic and inelastic scattering, single and multi photon fluorescence, second harmonic generation, etc. The most probable phenomena by far are light absorption and elastic scattering.

Light absorption happens when light of a particular energy level (characterized by its wavelength) stimulates the electron clouds of specific molecules to jump to a higher energy state and then gradually fall back to baseline transforming the light energy to heat. These molecules are called chromophores and in skin the major ones are melanin and hemoglobin (both the oxygenated and the deoxygenated type). If light is delivered to the tissue at a sufficient enough intensity, the generated heat following absorption can cause damage to the molecule. Such a process can be used for beneficial purposes such as the destruction of bilirubin in jaundiced infants, but it can also be the cause of unwanted phenomena such as alterations in the DNA molecules following UVR exposure.

Elastic light scattering occurs when the direction of light propagation is changed after light interacts with molecules or agglomerations of molecules. In skin tissue major light scattering centers are keratin fibrils, organelles (including nuclei and melanocytes), cell membranes, and in the dermis collagen and elastin fibers. Whereas light absorption is the reason that skin has color, elastic scattering is the reason why skin is not transparent. Together with absorption, light scattering is an important factor of determining the penetration depth that an incident light on the skin will reach before most of it will diffuse back out of the tissue. Thus they are both factors to be considered when trying to understand for example the extent of UVR-induced damage in the skin.

During the first months of life, infant skin has been known to have less constitutive pigmentation than adult skin, as well as minimal amounts of facultative pigmentation due to lack of previous exposure to the sun [1]. Moreover, recent work showing differences in papilla organization between infant and adult skin [2, 3] indicates differences in the vascular network at least at the capillary level. Therefore, both melanin (pigmentation) and hemoglobin (in the vasculature) concentrations and distributions differ between infant and adult, which points to differences in light absorption properties.

Light scattering properties are also expected to be different between infant and adult skin since: a) infant stratum corneum (SC) appears to be better hydrated than adult [2, 3], b) the structure of the epidermis is different (SC and supra-papillary epidermis are thicker in adult) [2, 3], and c) the structure of the dermal extracellular matrix are different (e.g. collagen fibers are thicker in adult skin [4]).

Taking all the above into account it is reasonable to conclude that since the optical properties between infant and adult skin are not the same, the intensity and extend of the effects following light-tissue interactions may also differ. For example, the relatively low amounts of melanin and SC scattering due to hydration in infants compared to adults suggest that infant skin may be unusually vulnerable to penetration and damage by incident UVR.

It is widely accepted that both cumulative and intermittent exposure to solar UVR are linked to a variety of deleterious outcomes such as sunburn, premature aging, and decreased immune functions. Compelling evidence has linked sun exposure in early childhood to skin cancer later in life as well [5-9]. At the same time, various environmental and cultural trends in the past few decades appear to have significantly increased exposure to UVR for children and adolescents in many parts of the world [5, 10-12]. While the projected risk of developing melanoma later in life was 1 in 1500 for newborns in 1935, recent estimates have elevated this risk currently to 1 in 33 [13]. Rates of all forms of skin cancer have been increasing worldwide, with an estimated 1,000,000 new cases of non-melanoma skin cancer and 60,000 new melanomas diagnosed in the U.S. alone in 2008 [14, 15]. Rates of nonmelanoma skin cancer in younger people appear to be rising as well, particularly among young women, although further studies are required to confirm [16].

These alarming trends and statistics have fueled considerable efforts over the past few decades to investigate the biologic effects of light. They have also transformed concerns about overexposure to solar radiation, particularly early in life, into major public health efforts promoting comprehensive sun protection for infants and children. These groups are particularly vulnerable considering the relatively lower levels of protective melanin and higher surface area-to-weight ratio compared to adults.

Despite these suspicions, very few existing studies have targeted the specific effects of light, including ultraviolet light, on infant skin. This lack of attention may be due, at least in part, to the fact that many of UVR-induced effects are not seen until adulthood. Most current knowledge of the UVR-induced effects on infant skin has been derived from extrapolating studies on adult skin and reflect a limited understanding of the way infant skin develops. In fact, until recently, the bulk of research about any form of light on infant skin has involved the blue-light phototherapy used to treat neonatal jaundice.

In the next chapters we begin by reviewing the risks involved with UVR exposure and examine the published literature on the effects of UVR on infant skin involving cell culture models, animal models, and human clinical trials. We then examine the better studied blue-light phototherapy and propose some ideas for future research in infant skin photobiology.

Chapter 2

RISKS ASSOCIATED WITH EXPOSURE OF SKIN TO UVR EARLY IN LIFE

This section reviews studies concerning risks of UVR exposure during infancy and childhood, as well as epidemiologic evidence showing alarmingly high rates of sun exposure and sunburn at these ages in many parts of the world. Overexposure to either UVA (320-400 nm) or UVB (290-320 nm) radiation at any age can seriously damage human skin. UVB radiation can cause acute inflammation, including sunburn, and has been strongly linked to the development of both basal and squamous cell carcinoma [17]. Once considered innocuous, UVA is now believed to accelerate the aging process as well as promote UVB-induced cancers by suppressing processes of the cutaneous immunity [14, 18]. Importantly, evidence from case control and other epidemiologic studies has highlighted the particularly serious, long-term consequences of overexposure in infancy and childhood. This evidence includes studies linking intense exposure to UVR and sunburn during childhood to increased risks of developing cutaneous malignant melanoma (CMM) [15, 19-21] and basal cell carcinoma (BCC) [22, 23] later in life, as well as studies linking exposure to UVR over longer periods of time to the development of squamous cell carcinoma (SCC) [17, 24]. Sunlight, in fact, remains the only environmental factor definitively linked to both melanocytic nevi and cutaneous melanoma [25-28].

Concerns about long-term health effects of early sun exposure have prompted public health organizations worldwide to issue comprehensive sun protection recommendations to screen or block UVR exposure with particular emphasis on infants and children. Recommended practices include sun avoidance as a first-line strategy for infants less than six months of age, as well as wearing hats, tightly woven clothing, and sunglasses when sun avoidance is not an option. Children and infants above six months of age are also advised to use topical sunscreen products of SPF 30 or higher, regardless of skin type [29-33].

2.1. CUTANEOUS MELANOCYTIC MELANOMA

While malignant melanoma accounts for only 4% of all skin cancers worldwide, it is associated with approximately 75% of skin cancer-related deaths [34]. While cutaneous melanoma is rare in infants and children, prognosis and response to this malignancy in the pediatric population resembles those seen in adults [35, 36]. In addition, excessive sun exposure and/or a history of blistering sunburns in early childhood is an established risk factor for developing malignant melanoma later in life [37-39]. Fair skin, blue eyes, and red or blond hair are additional risk factors, as is a history of immunosuppression, a family or personal history of melanoma, or having xeroderma pigmentosum or atypical ("dysplastic") nevi. An estimated 50-65% of all malignant melanoma arises in pre-existing nevi [40].

The exact relationship between childhood sun exposure and the lifetime risk of developing CMM remains controversial. Intermittent, or recreational, sun exposure, during childhood has been hypothesized to be the major cause of CMM, and numerous case-control studies with adults have shown an association between the number and severity of childhood sunburns and the risk of developing this skin cancer [1, 15, 35-38, 41, 42]. In the Nurses' Health Study, blistering sunburns at 15 to 20 years of age were significantly associated with increased risk of developing CMM (relative risk, 2.2 for >5 sunburns vs. none) [39]. However, the time-course involved, the need for retrospective analysis, and variant measures of childhood sun exposure across studies make it difficult to determine the exact relationship between childhood sun exposure and melanoma [23, 26, 43].

Ecological studies assessing ambient sun exposure appear to be more accurate and consistent than case-control studies in determining effects of exposure to sunlight during specific age periods. A systematic review of the literature using computerized bibliographic databases and article reference lists found that such studies consistently reported lower risks of melanoma among people who resided in low UVR environments in childhood than in those who resided at high UVR environments [44]. These findings are consistent with earlier studies on migrants to Israel and Australia suggesting that intense sun exposure in early childhood may be more important in increasing the risk of cutaneous melanoma in adulthood than cumulative years of sun exposure [45, 46]. Suggestions have also been made that melanocytes in early life may be more sensitive to the sun, resulting in changes in DNA that may lead to the formation of unstable and pre-malignant moles [30]. However, adult exposure to sun also appears to play a role in increasing the risk of melanoma, and whether early childhood is a critical period in which melanocytes are particularly susceptible to the biological effects of sunlight remains a subject of controversy [47, 48].

What is clear is that avoiding harmful UVR exposure in youth appears to reduce melanoma risk more than similar avoidance in adulthood [49]. This may be related to the fact that child and adolescent behavior patterns may intensify UVR exposure and blistering sunburns. Infants also have not experienced the gradual exposure to UVR that stimulates facultative pigmentation and thus may be more susceptible to the damaging effects of excessive exposure to sunlight [1]. Several recent epidemiologic studies have suggested an association between early-life UVR exposure and specific somatic mutations at specific body sites. Intensive, intermittent UVR exposure is frequently linked to melanomas on the trunk, for example, whereas chronic UVR exposure seems more frequently linked to melanomas on the head [42, 43, 50]. Childhood exposure to UVR has also been linked to specific types of genetic damage. One population-based case study associated high exposure to ambient UVR at ages 0-20 years with *BRAF* mutations and a mean age of melanoma diagnosis of 47.3, and high UVR exposure at ages 50-60 years with *NRAS* mutations and a mean age of diagnosis of 62.1 years [51]. While these studies reflect broad population trends and require additional confirmation, they suggest significant differences between the response of infant and adult skin to UVR.

2.2. MELANOCYTIC NEVI

Melanocytic nevi (MN), common skin neoplasms thought to be slightly altered melanocytes, can be either congenital or acquired. Most acquired MN appear after infancy, with numbers and size increasing throughout early childhood and peaking in young adulthood. MN in infants and children are primarily of concern because a small percentage of them may eventually transform into cutaneous melanoma. Strong epidemiologic evidence links the total number of benign MN on the body to the development of cutaneous melanoma [52-55] and some nevi appear to be precursor lesions to melanomas [56]. Thus, acquired MN should be closely monitored for atypical features suggestive of malignant changes.

Very few studies to date have looked at the development of nevi in the first few years of life, although there is strong evidence that risk is closely related to cumulative exposure to UVR and that density of nevi is correlated with total sun exposure [26, 29, 57-60]. A study in Queensland, Australia, where one finds the highest rate of melanoma in the world as well as the highest numbers of melanocytic nevi among children, associated both acute and chronic sun exposure in children to the development of these nevi [25]. Another study of Australian preschoolers also found that the number of lifetime sunburns and the severity of sunburns were significantly related to the presence of large acquired MN [61].

Accumulating evidence suggests that mild to moderate sun exposure, even without sunburn, is sufficient to induce MN in children, particularly in those with light skin color, blond or red hair, and blue eyes and/or whose parents had large numbers of moles. A recent cluster prevalence study in Queensland, Australia involving toddlers (ages 1-3), for example, associated the many MN that developed at a very young age with heavy sun exposure and with freckling, as well as with Caucasian ethnicity. Conversely, toddlers who were protected from the sun, whether through dark skin color, tanning ability, or the frequent application of sunscreen, showed relatively low nevi counts, and those who wore hats had lower nevi counts on the face but not on other body sites [62]. Consistent with these findings was a study of German nursery school children showing that moderate sun exposure without sunburns, such as outdoor activities during a German summer, induced nevus development. This same study found a strong association between nevus development in children and the number of moles in their parents, as well as a direct relationship between the cumulative duration of sun exposure and the risk of developing MN [63]. While all of these findings stem from studies of toddlers rather than infants specifically, they suggest that in very young children sun exposure, even without burning, may be sufficient to increase risk of MN and, ultimately, cutaneous melanoma and that exposure to UVR below the threshold of sunburn may substantially damage DNA and precipitate malignant transformation in keratinocytes and melanocytes [58].

Sunburns on the other hand, do seem to increase the risk of large MN. Estimating the erythemally effective dose of solar UVR from questionnaire data combined with local UVR biometry, a study of preschool children in Townsville, Australia found that lifetime number of sunburns and the severity of sunburns were significantly related to the presence of large acquired MN during follow-up. The same study found that total number of hours of sun exposure and tendency to burn were independent risk factors for MN [61]. In addition, a small study recently suggested that nevi acquired on sun-exposed skin during childhood and adolescence are genetically distinct from congenital nevi. This study analyzed the mutation spectrum of congenital nevi to see if it differed from that of the MN that develop on sun-exposed skin during childhood and adolescence, which are known to harbor *BRAF* mutations more frequently than *NRAS* mutations. The congenital nevi, though indistinguishable histopathologically, showed no *BRAF* mutations, but 81% (26/32) had mutations in *NRAS* [64].

2.3. NONMELANOMA SKIN CANCER

Of the 1 million skin cancers diagnosed annually in the United States, approximately 75-80% are basal cell carcinomas (BCC) and 15-20% are squamous cell carcinomas (SCC) [11, 12]. BCC is a malignant neoplasm originating at the basal layer of the epidermis. While it rarely metastasizes, untreated BCC can invade local tissue and eventually lead to extensive functional and cosmetic damage. Cutaneous SCC develops in the epidermis, usually from precursor lesions called solar or actinic keratosis. Some forms of SCC are superficially invasive and can be easily treated before causing disfiguring tissue loss, while more aggressive types carry significant risk of metastasis and life-threatening complications.

BCC rarely occurs in children unless they have an underlying genetic condition [65], but intensive UVR exposure in childhood and adolescence can underlie development of BCC later in life [66]. One population-based case-control study showed a significantly increased risk of BCC in men who had had relatively high levels of recreational sunlight exposure in adolescence and childhood (ages 0 to 19 years), with the relationship most pronounced among sun-sensitive subjects whose skin tended to burn rather than tan. This study found no association between cumulative sun exposure and BCC, consistent with results from a population-based, case-control study in Western Australia suggesting that a particular amount of sun exposure delivered in infrequent, intense increments increases BCC risk more than similar doses of UVR delivered more continuously over the same period of time [8, 67].

In contrast, the bulk of evidence suggests that cumulative exposure to UVR over a lifetime is a significant risk factor for SCC, regardless of age or pattern of exposure [68]. While SCC rarely develops in children without a predisposing condition such as xeroderma pigmentosum, human papilloma virus infection, or immunosuppression [40], chronic exposures to sunlight in the first decades of life is associated with the development of SCC in adulthood [66].

Exposure to UVR in infancy and early childhood can also promote the development of solar keratoses, suggesting, by implication, that reducing exposure to sunlight in childhood may substantially reduce long-term risk of developing SCC [69]. In a study comparing Australian-born adults to Australian adults who had migrated from Great Britain at various ages (both groups of Caucasian ancestry), the proportion of persons with solar keratoses in the group who arrived as adults never reached the proportion found in Australian natives. The randomization of the 588 subjects enrolled in the study was stratified according to sex and self-rated skin type (burn only and never tan, burn first and then tan, or tan only and never burn). Younger persons in the group of immigrants who arrived in Australia between the ages of 1 and 20 years also had a lower proportion of solar keratoses than native-born Australian adults, while their older peers had the same or even higher proportion [70]. Regular sunscreen use has also been shown to prevent solar keratoses and by implication reduce the risk of developing SCC [57].

Chapter 3

EFFECTS OF UVR
ON THE BIOLOGY OF
INFANT SKIN

Thus far we examined the risks associated with exposure to UVR early in life. We will now turn our attention to the possible mechanisms that could be responsible for the existence of such risks.

The effects of exposure to solar UVR on adult skin are well recognized and include erythema, hyper-pigmentation, local immunosuppression, and long-term risks of photoaging and skin cancer [71-75]. UVR has the ability to alter the skin microenvironment and has long been associated with suppression of the skin immune system (SIS) and an altered balance between epidermal proliferation and differentiation [76, 77]. In addition, it is widely recognized that exposure to UVB directly damages DNA and potentially facilitates the development of skin cancer [78-80]. However, until recently attempts to elucidate and quantify these effects in infants and children have been undermined by a number of technical limitations, namely a lack of in vivo methods appropriate for use in very young subjects [8, 67, 81-83]. As a result, the bulk of the current understanding of UVR effects on the biology of infant skin comes from studies using either animal models or cell cultures. However, the advent of several new non-invasive measurement techniques in the past few years has allowed for some illuminating insights from human clinical trials investigating the response of infant skin to UVR.

3.1. CELL AND TISSUE CULTURE MODELS

3.1.1. DNA Repair Response and Cutaneous Immunity

Early studies of cultured human epidermal keratinocytes showed no significant age-related differences in the rate and extent of repair or normal replication of DNA after either intense or chronic, low-level UVR exposure [84, 85]. However, considerable evidence suggests that early sun exposure may predispose cells to impaired DNA repair capacity later in life. In a recent study, for example, cultured human keratinocytes derived from newborn, young adult, and older adult donors were exposed to a single physiologic dose of solar-simulated radiation (SSR). Effects of the exposure were analyzed on genes previously associated with UVR modulation in newborn keratinocytes, cytokines implicated in UVR immunomodulatory effects, and a recently cloned gene (*SPR2*) known to be induced during keratinocyte differentiation and by lethal UVC (100-290 nm) irradiation. Although age had relatively little effect on the response to UVR, the combination of aging and SSR exposure ("photoaging") markedly increased the inducibility of the oncogene c-fos and decreased the baseline expression of *SPR2* and IL-1ra relative to cells from sun-protected skin of the same donors. These findings may help explain the predisposition to photocarcinogenesis in photoaged, as opposed to infant and otherwise unexposed, skin [86]. A subsequent study of DNA repair capacity of skin fibroblasts suggests that this age-related reduction in DNA repair synthesis following UVR exposure may be due to decreased expression of genes involved in nucleotide excision repair (NER) [87].

Growing evidence from proteomic studies also suggests that unique features of the skin immune system may alter the effect of UVR on infant skin. The concept of the SIS reflects current understanding of the skin's ability to protect against penetration by external agents not just by physical means but also through cellular immunologic mechanisms. The SIS response can involve either an active immune response or an induced tolerance, both of which vary with the preexisting cellular microenvironment. Cutaneous immune reactions include responses by dendritic antigen-presenting cells such as Langerhans cells (LC), monocytes/macrophages, mast cells, lymphatic/vascular endothelial cells, and T lymphocytes, as well as humoral components such as cytokines, neuropeptides, prostaglandins, and free radicals [88]. LC are a type of immune-system-activating dendritic cells in the skin, thought to help alert the system to the presence of foreign pathogens and other foreign materials (although some evidence suggests that they may actually dampen the skin reaction to infection and inflammation) [89]. Normally neonates have a relatively small number and density of LC, and these cells have relatively short dendrites and few receptor molecules critical for immune response. LC density, distribution, morphology, and cell marker expression gradually change over time [88, 90-92].

Recent findings from proteomic studies comparing neonatal and adult murine tissue have identified numerous proteins uniquely expressed in neonatal skin that may influence the development of the skin immune system and, by implication, the impact of UVR on infant skin. These proteins include Stefin A, which appears to decrease with age and may play a role in promoting cellular proliferation in neonatal skin as well as abnormal proliferative conditions [88]. Similarly, the peroxiredoxins, which play a protective role against oxidative damage, appear to be expressed at greater levels in neonatal skin. Recent findings that peroxiredoxin-2 may be involved in inhibiting T lymphocytes and dendritic cells suggest that this protein may also be an important regulatory factor in the developing SIS [88, 93]. Such differences between the developing and the developed SIS may point in the future to differences in UVR-induced immune-modulation between infant and adult skin.

3.1.2. UVB-Induced Vitamin D Production

Accumulating *in vitro* evidence supports the concept that UVB-induced Vitamin D production within the skin may help modulate the development of the infant SIS [88]. UVB converts 7-dehydrocholesterol in the skin to previtamin D3, which is rapidly transformed into vitamin D3 and then hydroxylated in the liver, kidney, and other tissues, including the keratinocytes, into its biologically active form, the hormone calcitriol (1,25(OH)2D3) [94-99]. Critically important in the maintenance of healthy bones as well as in cell growth, calcitriol has well-known anti-proliferative and pro-differentiating effects and has long been known to influence the differentiation, maturation, and survival of dendritic cells. It also appears to affect the cutaneous immune response by acting directly on cells that express the vitamin D receptor such as keratinocytes, LCs, $\gamma\delta$ T cells, mast cells, dermal dendritic cells, and macrophages [100, 101] and by indirectly altering the production of immunomodulatory cytokines and growth factors by keratinocytes [88].

Evidence from cell and tissue culture studies suggests that calcitriol may play a role in dampening the neonatal immune response by acting directly on cells within the SIS that express vitamin D receptor, as well as suppressing production of immunomodulatory cytokines and growth factors by keratinocytes [88, 100, 101]. Adding calcitriol to highly enriched LC populations from adult mice inhibits stimulation of allogeneic T cells [102, 103] and alters production of inflammatory cytokines and chemokines, stimulating production of IL-1β, CCL3, CCL4 and CCL5 as well as Th1-type chemokines (CXCL9, CXCL10, and CXCL11) and inhibiting production of Th2-type chemokines (CL17 and CCL22) [104]. In addition, calcitriol inhibits the maturation of LC, possibly by inhibiting the alloantigen-stimulation of naïve T cells [105].

At the same time, other *in vitro* studies suggest that calcitriol may also help protect keratinocytes from UVR-induced apoptosis, although the way these effects manifest themselves in neonatal skin specifically has not yet been explored. Consistent with findings from animal studies, calcitriol and related compounds have been shown to reduce and help repair UVB-induced cyclobutane pyrimidine dimers in cultures of irradiated human skin cells, thereby contributing to the prevention of mutations and apoptosis [106].

3.2. ANIMAL MODELS

3.2.1. Modulation of the Skin Immune System

Numerous studies using murine models have confirmed that intense sun exposure early in life is one of many external agents that can alter the SIS. Current understanding of the UVR impact on the SIS has been built upon the pioneering studies establishing that the primary molecular event in generating the systemic immunosuppression by UVR in skin of mice is the formation of pyrimidine dimers [80]. This work demonstrated that alterations to the skin environment by either UVR or chemical carcinogens set off cellular events that ultimately suppress T cell generation that might otherwise inhibit the development of antigenic tumors [107]. These findings are consistent with retrospective, epidemiologic data showing that immunologic events in infancy can have profound effects in adulthood, and particularly those studies linking intense, intermittent exposure of skin to UVR in early childhood to CMM later in life.

SIS development and its response to UVR are little understood in humans. However, numerous studies using animal models suggest that UVR can profoundly change the neonatal immune system, including suppressing both innate and adaptive immune responses and predisposing cells to subsequent carcinogenic changes. Various studies of transgenic mice indicate that both single high-dose and chronic exposure to SSR in early life may compromise the development of the SIS, potentially increasing the risk of developing UVR-related cancers [71, 88, 108, 109].

Although the long-term implications of neonatal exposure to UVR remain unclear, both repeated and chronic doses of SSR have been shown to reduce the number of LC in the epidermis and increase the number of dendritic cells in lymph nodes that drain irradiated skin sites [109]. Subsequent work, however, has suggested that although single, high-dose UVB exposure in neonatal mice alters the development of neonatal LC to produce a short-term reduction in their number, it enhances immune response at maturity. In one study the reduction in LC density among neonatal mice exposed to high doses (2 kJ/m/s) of UVB radiation was substantially greater than in equivalently exposed older mice, although at lower doses there were no differences in susceptibility. However, at maturity, the mice irradiated as neonates showed an increased ability to respond to topically applied antigen: they transported more antigen to the lymph nodes, and their lymph node dendritic cells showed an enhanced ability to stimulate T-cell proliferation, with the response skewed towards a Th2 type response [71]. Elucidating the precise characteristics of the skin in neonatal mice that underlie this apparent sensitivity to UVR will require additional investigation.

3.2.2. Implications for Carcinogenesis

It has been suggested that the lack of an acute inflammatory response in neonatal mice (e.g. lack of neutrophil tissue infiltration, vascular dilatation, increased vascular permeability, and release of inflammatory mediators) may promote tolerance and limit immune development in neonatal skin, potentially increasing susceptibility of neonatal mice to carcinogenic changes [72, 73, 88]. An alternative hypothesis is that neonatal mice may be particularly susceptible to the UVR-induced melanoma due to retention of UVR-related damage by their abundant immature melanocytes [72].

Various studies suggest that melanoma antigens generated during the neonatal period are likely to generate long-lived, antigen-specific regulatory T cells that may eventually undermine effective anti-tumor immunity. Exposing the skin of neonatal mice to UVR, even with a single high dose, appears to alter the microenvironment. Mildly erythemal doses of UVR in the neonatal period have been shown to alter the immune environment to favor antigen-specific immune suppression and skin tumor development, including a gradual increase in the number of regulatory T cells and B cells in the local lymph nodes that becomes significant by adulthood [71, 88]. Together with the immunosuppression linked to intense UVB exposure and the propensity of neonatal skin to develop tolerance, these changes may increase the risk of developing skin cancer, particularly melanoma later in life [88].

Although the induction of melanoma is a multi-factorial process, work by Noonan et al. using UV-irradiated HGF/SF transgenic models have provided specific experimental support for neonatal melanoma susceptibility, as well as direct evidence that neonatal UVB is responsible for inducing cutaneous melanoma [108]. Studies using a genetically engineered mouse model have shown that single high-dose exposures to UVB, but not UVA, can cause a tumor reminiscent of human melanoma in neonatal animals, but not in adults [74, 108]. In addition, several studies using transgenic mouse models have shown that a single dose of UVR is sufficient to induce melanoma in neonatal mice carrying specific mutations (*Ras* or *HGF/SF*) [75, 110-115]. Consistent with these findings are studies of young, transgenic mice showing that UVB can promote the induction of cutaneous melanoma, as well as serve as a cofactor promoting the growth of melanoma induced by chemical agents [115].

A recent study also suggests that neonatal melanocytes exposed to UVR are unusually sensitive to UVR-induced proliferation and transformation [116]. Known to inhibit apoptosis, increase melanin production, and enhance DNA repair, the activation of melanocytes is a well-recognized protective response to sun exposure in mammals, including humans. Dendritic processes transport melanosomes from the melanocyte cell body to the dendritic tips and then to keratinocytes [117]. Melanocytes in neonatal mice, in contrast to those from older mice, migrate to the epidermal basal layer following a single dose of UVR, apparently relocating from the outer root sheath of the hair follicle, with numbers peaking 3-5 days after exposure [116, 118-120]. Moreover, in melanoma-prone mice with melanocyte-specific over-expression of *HrasG12V*, these basal layer melanocytes were larger and had more dendritic processes than those of UVR-treated wild-type mice. As the proliferation of melanocytes in response to sun damage may play a role in increasing the risk of malignant melanoma [121-123], these findings support the concept of an unusual degree of sensitivity to UVR in neonatal mouse melanocytes and may help explain the efficacy of UVR to induce melanoma in mice carrying oncogenic mutations.

3.2.3. UVB-Induced Vitamin D Production

Numerous studies using animal models suggest that UVR-induced vitamin D may serve as an immune modulator and that the direct action of calcitriol (the active form of vitamin D in the body) on the production of immunomodulatory molecules by keratinocytes may be distinctive in early life. On the one hand, topical application of a vitamin D analog to human [102] and of calcitriol to mouse skin [103] has been shown to cause significant immunosuppression to a contact sensitizer, presumably due to reduced LC function. At the same time, other studies suggest that calcitriol and related compounds may reduce UVB-induced cyclobutane pyrimidine dimers within keratinocytes [124]. They may also help promote efficient repair of UVB-induced cyclobutane pyrimidine dimers by inducing the formation of metallothionein, an antioxidant found in human skin after UVB exposure and believed necessary to prevent keratinocyte apoptosis [125, 126]. It remains unclear whether the higher levels of calcitriol produced in response to UVR by children skin [127] specifically modulate the function of dendritic cells or repair UVB-induced DNA damage associated with increased skin cancer risk. Still, preliminary data suggest that adding vitamin D3 to the diet may reduce UVB-induced DNA damage in female, but not male, mice during the neonatal period [88].

3.3. HUMAN STUDIES

3.3.1. Developing Barrier Properties

Recent studies confirming and elucidating differences between the barrier properties of infant and adult skin have contributed to the notion that newborn skin may be particularly vulnerable to UVR. These findings build on existing knowledge that infant skin has a significantly thinner SC than adult, as well as relatively limited melanin production, and lack of prior facultative pigmentation [128-133] and suggest that these differences continue far longer than previous believed. Consisting of layers of flattened non-nucleated keratinized cells, the SC regulates trans-epidermal water loss (TEWL), which has been used extensively as an indicator of barrier function [128-130, 134, 135]. The natural barrier protection from the aqueous intra-uterine environment provided to the fetus by the *vernix caseosa* is wiped away at birth, leaving protection from external agents in the terrestrial environment to the SC. The contribution of the SC to the protection against UVR can be considered from the point of limiting UVR penetration due to its light scattering properties as well as absorption of UVR by SC molecules such as urocanic acid [136].

There is not a lot of information about how this physical and immunologic barrier protection develops after the first month of life. In contrast to the relatively steady state of adult skin, neonatal skin has been shown repeatedly to adjust its thickness, pH, and hydration to various environmental conditions during the first month of life [132, 137-141]. However, recent *in vivo* studies using non-invasive methodologies suggest that the skin maturation process in human continues far longer than the neonatal period, potentially leaving the skin particularly vulnerable to the effects of UVR throughout infancy and even into toddlerhood. Ultrastructural and morphometrical evaluations of normal dermal connective tissue have established that dermal constituents such as collagen, elastin fibers, and mesenchymal cells change substantially during the perinatal period, underlying corresponding changes in the extracellular matrix during this time period as well [142]. A recent study of babies ages 3-24 months and their mothers using non-invasive microscopy tools showed significant differences in morphologic features of the SC, including glyph density and dermal papillae size, density, and distribution, as well as the ratio between visible surface papillae and glyphs [3]. The SC and total epidermis were significantly thinner in the infants. In addition, granular cells were significantly smaller and denser, and corneocytes significantly smaller, on the upper inner arms, outer forearms, and legs of the infants, indicating faster turnover rate and greater surface area for increased absorption. Also suggestive of a relatively thinner and vulnerable SC in infants are reports of *in vivo* Fourier-transform infrared spectroscopy and diffuse reflectance spectroscopy documenting significantly fewer total lipids and sebaceous lipids in infant skin, as well as relatively lower concentrations of melanin (authors' unpublished data).

These findings are consistent with new evidence suggesting that infant skin continues to develop far longer than the first month of life. One recent prospective, cohort study, for example, showed no difference in either initial skin appearance or biophysical measurements (TEWL and surface hydration) between infants who went on to develop atopic dermatitis and those who remained lesion-free, suggesting that barrier impairment found in atopic dermatitis, rather than being inherent, may be secondary to dermatitic skin changes long after the neonatal period [143]. Infants aged 8-24 months have also been shown to have significantly higher skin capacitance and pH values on both the skin of the ventral forearm and buttocks than adults [141].

Both barrier function and water handling properties of the SC also appear to continue to develop well beyond the first month of life and at least as long as the first year. These properties are influenced by a complex interplay of factors, including the presence of natural moisturizing factor (NMF), corneocyte maturity/hydrophilicity, lipid quantity and phase, density of appendages, surface microrelief, and diffusion path length [2]. Earlier evidence based primarily on TEWL measurements suggested that the SC barrier is fully functional at birth [128, 129, 132, 139, 144, 145]. However, the conclusion that term infants are born with a functionally mature SC, as well as the wide variations in the measured TEWL values of these earlier studies, may reflect differences in environmental acclimation times, number and age range of subjects, body site studied, or the type of measurement instruments used – particularly the use of open chamber instruments, which tend to report TEWL values in the skin of term infants lower than or equal to those reported from adults [128, 129, 144]. Our more recent work including *in vivo* Raman confocal microspectroscopy in infants gives consistently higher values for skin water concentration and water absorption-desorption rates in the SC of infants versus adults. Applied for the first time on infant skin, this technique allows the acquisition of Raman spectra as a function of skin depth with a lateral resolution of 1 μm (x and y directions) and a depth resolution of 5 μm (z direction). These data can then be analyzed for water content, and water concentration profiles, calculated as a function of skin depth. Findings from this study are in agreement with some published reports from term infants [130, 145] and support the notion that although the SC may appear to be intact shortly after birth, it develops adult-like water handling properties and associated protective barrier properties only after the first year of life [2].

Additional studies have suggested that both water content and water concentration in the skin remain relatively high throughout at least the first year of life. Previous studies have suggested that SC hydration is low at birth and increases with postnatal age [130, 132, 133, 137, 141], with duration of the SC hydration increase ranging from two weeks postpartum [132] to 30–90 days postpartum [133]. Measurements of skin conductance and water distribution obtained using *in vivo* Raman confocal microspectroscopy indicates that this process may continue throughout the first year and that infant SC is significantly more hydrated than adult SC throughout this period. In this study, infants aged 3-33 months had more water throughout most parts of the SC on the lower ventral surfaces of their arms than did adults. The epidermis of infants aged 3-12 months had a steeper water gradient and higher water concentration than that of adults within the top 20 μm. Infant skin also had a significantly lower concentration of NMF in the first 12 μm [2]. These lower relative NMF concentrations may themselves impair barrier function and increase water desorption, since NMF plays a key role in maintaining skin hydration by absorbing and retaining water.

The signs of functional immaturity throughout the first year of life suggest increased vulnerability of infant skin to external influences, potentially including UVR. Such differences between adult and infant skin in SC water content influence skin surface morphology, the desquamation process, and epidermal expression of keratins and other proteins and thus may compromise barrier integrity [146-151]. The specific effects of this increased water content on skin optics and UVR penetration remain to be determined. In addition, the fact that dermal scatter of light is known to be greater in dry than in well-hydrated SC suggests that the increased water content found in infant skin may allow relatively more UVR to penetrate it.

3.3.2. Melanogenesis: Developing Skin Response to UVR

Preliminary *in vivo* studies using non-invasive methods suggest that skin response to solar UVR in infants may begin as early as the first summer of life. A recent longitudinal study that we performed demonstrated increases in facultative pigmentation in infants in the first and second summers of life as well as for their mothers [152]. In this study we compared skin changes over time in healthy Caucasian infants and their mothers using diffuse reflectance spectroscopy to measure the apparent concentrations of skin chromophores (melanin, oxy-hemoglobin, and deoxy-hemoglobin). All groups experienced increases of similar magnitude in apparent concentration of melanin on exposed skin sites (dorsal forearm) compared to unexposed skin sites (upper inner arm) over the summer months. While pigmentation normally increases in the first years of life [138, 153-155] and itself plays a role in sun protection, the fact that such increases happen as early as the first summer raise concerns, especially given the association between rapid melanogenesis and UVR-induced DNA damage [156]. Although these findings require confirmation, they suggest that incidental UVR exposure and the associated photodamage may begin as early as the first summer of life, before the physical and immunologic barrier reaches maturity.

3.3.3. UVB Exposure and
Vitamin D Requirements

Mounting evidence suggests that many adults and children around the world are vitamin D deficient [157-172]. Coupled with extensive evidence linking vitamin D deficiency to a broad spectrum of diseases, including various cancers, these findings have raised concerns about recent efforts to limit UVR exposure in infants and children. Over 12% of the 380 healthy infants and toddlers recently examined in an urban primary care clinic were found to have vitamin D deficiency (< 20 ng/mL) and 40% had levels below an accepted optimal threshold (<30 ng/mL) regardless of age or degree of skin pigmentation [173]. Some dermatologists have also expressed concerns that sun protective measures may restrict vitamin D3 production in the skin, which is normally the body's primary source of the vitamin. As a result, there is still considerable debate among dermatologists, about the relative risks and benefits of sun exposure, oral vitamin D supplementation, and the precise amount of sunlight exposure required to balance its risks and benefits [19, 49, 70, 156, 174-176].

Complicating efforts to resolve this debate are the many factors influencing vitamin D synthesis in the skin, particularly the amount of skin pigmentation but also body mass, amount of exposed skin and unprotected skin, season, latitude, and air pollution levels [177-180]. In addition, recent evidence suggests variable responsiveness to UVB radiation among individuals, as well as low vitamin D status among some individuals despite abundant sun exposure [181]. Nonetheless, the vast majority of dermatologists and pediatricians today believe that existing evidence still supports the comprehensive sun protection measures advocated by the American Academy of Pediatrics (AAP), including sun avoidance for infants under 6 months of age and sun protection measures such as protective clothing and sunscreen when sun avoidance is impossible, together with a minimum daily vitamin D intake of 400 IU for all infants and children beginning soon after birth [30, 97].

Chapter 4

BLUE LIGHT PHOTOTHERAPY
FOR JAUNDICE

In contrast to UVR, the effects of exposure to blue light on infant skin have been extensively investigated, largely due to the widespread use of phototherapy to treat neonatal jaundice. An estimated 60% of normal newborns develop jaundice, a yellow discoloration of the skin and sclera, within the first week of life. This condition is due to excessive conjugated bilirubin (hyperbilirubinemia) that results from excessive bilirubin formation, coupled with the inability of the neonatal liver to clear it rapidly enough from the blood. In most infants jaundice is a normal and transient development that resolves without medical treatment, but in some infants extremely high levels of unconjugated bilirubin if left untreated can lead to bilirubin encephalopathy and subsequent kernicterus, a chronic form of bilirubin encephalopathy that can result in permanent, debilitating neurodevelopmental handicaps or even death. Consequently, newborns are routinely monitored for jaundice and treated with phototherapy when total serum levels of bilirubin exceed those specified by AAP guidelines [24]. Such treatment is designed to lower the concentration of circulating bilirubin and to keep it from increasing. The AAP also recommends prophylactic phototherapy for infants with low birth weight or early gestational age [182].

During phototherapy, absorbed light energy transformed to heat changes the shape and structure of bilirubin so that it will be excreted even without conjugation. Following phototherapy treatment the skin no longer looks jaundiced. Dermal and subcutaneous bilirubin absorb the light, inducing several different photochemical reactions that rapidly generate yellow stereoisomers of bilirubin as well as various lower molecular weight, colorless derivatives. These photoisomers have also been found in the blood of adults after sunbathing [183, 184]. Several efforts have been made to measure and characterize the photoisomers generated by intensive phototherapy, but further work must be done to elucidate their precise contributions of their specific photochemical pathway to eliminating bilirubin [183, 185, 186].

Bilirubin absorbs light most strongly in the blue region of the spectrum, and the generation rate of bilirubin photoproducts depends highly on light intensity and wavelength. In addition, tissue penetration increases greatly with increasing wavelength. As a result, the most effective wavelengths of light for treating neonatal jaundice appear to fall into the 460-490 nm range. UVR exposure is not generally a concern, since the phototherapy light sources used today do not emit significant amounts of erythemal UVR [183].

Although numerous clinical trials earlier in the 20th century established the efficacy of phototherapy in treating neonatal jaundice, ethical considerations preclude conducting any placebo-controlled trials to test the efficacy of the relatively high light doses used today, which in intensive therapy deliver irradiance of ≥ 30 $\mu W/cm^2/nm$ in the blue spectrum delivered to the maximum surface area [183]. There is considerably more evidence, however, about adverse effects of intensive phototherapy on infant skin. While reports of clinically significant toxicity are rare, the skin, serum, and urine of infants with cholestasis sometimes develop a dark, grayish-brown discoloration, a phenomenon known as "bronze baby syndrome" [187, 188]. This discoloration is thought to be due to the formation of a photo-oxidation product of bilirubin or to copper-bound porphyrins [189, 190], with possible contribution of biliverdin pigments [191] and disappears without significant sequelae once phototherapy concludes.

Phototherapy-induced erythematous and vesiculo-bullous eruptions have also been seen in newborns who were exposed to methylene blue prenatally or who are receiving agents such as frusemide or fluorescein dye for radiologic procedures [192-194]. More rarely, infants with severe cholestatic jaundice develop distinctive cutaneous complications. Several researchers, for example, have reported purpuric and bullous eruptions in neonates receiving phototherapy for hyperbilirubinemia, possibly from sensitization by accumulating porphyrins [195-197]. In fact, congenital porphyria should be considered in any infant who develops severe blistering during phototherapy. In addition, phototherapy is contraindicated for infants with congenital porphyria or a family history of porphyria, as well as in any infant receiving photosensitizing drugs. This may include infants treated with tin-mesoporpryrin, a drug currently being used experimentally to prevent and treat hyperbilirubinemia, some of whom have shown to develop erythematous rashes when exposed to sunlight or daylight fluorescent bulbs [183, 198].

A few studies have suggested that by acutely changing the infant's thermal environment, phototherapy can increase peripheral blood flow and thus produce insensible water loss. In one study, TEWL and skin hydration were measured in seven body areas before and during phototherapy in 31 preterm infants (25-36 weeks gestation) and found a mean increase of 26.4% in TEWL during phototherapy, particularly in the cubital fossa (45.9%), groin (35.4%), and back (29%). However, this study showed no significant differences in SC hydration in six of the seven body areas, either before or during phototherapy [199, 200]. The implications of these findings for fluid replacement in infants undergoing phototherapy and their relevance to phototherapy with relative low-heat light emitting diode sources remain to be determined [183].

Finally, there is still some controversy regarding the role that blue-light phototherapy may play in increasing the risk of developing atypical nevi in childhood, widely considered to be an important risk factors for melanoma later in life. In 2002-3 Csozma, Hencz, and Orvos studied 747 schoolchildren (14-18 years of age), nearly half of whom had received phototherapy to treat neonatal jaundice, to determine the prevalence of both common and atypical MN. They focused their study on adolescents because this is the age at which dysplastic nevi often develop. Although prevalence of common MN was similar in treated and untreated children, those who had received neonatal phototherapy were more likely to have multiple (>100) moles. In addition, neonatal blue-light phototherapy was associated with a significantly higher percentage of atypical nevi [201]. These results were consistent with a case-control prospective study that found significantly more large (2-5 mm diameter) nevi in children who had received intensive neonatal phototherapy than in a control group who had not [202]. These findings contrast with those of Bauer et al., who had earlier reported no association between neonatal treatment with a blue-light lamp and an increased risk of developing MN in younger children (ages 2 to 7 years) [203]. However, in a recent multicenter study with 828 nine-year-old children, over 22% of whom had received neonatal phototherapy, no evidence was found for a major role of blue-light phototherapy on subsequent nevus count regardless of the location or size of the nevi or the phototype of the child. In contrast, nevus count correlated with a light phototype, skin and hair color, blue/green eyes, and history of sunburn [204]. Some of the apparent contradictions between these studies may be related to the ages of children studied, since common MN generally first appear in early childhood, while dysplastic nevi tend to develop around puberty [201].

Chapter 5

CONCLUSION AND AREAS FOR FUTURE RESEARCH

Substantial epidemiologic evidence, coupled with accumulating experimental data from cell culture, animal models, and human studies, suggests that infant skin has a distinctive response to light, particularly UVR, and that this distinct response may make it particularly vulnerable to long-term photodamage. However, substantial gaps remain in the understanding of these effects from both epidemiologic and biologic perspectives. Even our considerable knowledge of the effects of intense blue light on infant skin being treated for jaundice leaves open fundamental questions at the molecular level that await answers from studies involving infant skin cell culture and animal models.

Future experimental research will be needed to identify and quantify changes in the epidermal microenvironment and SIS during the neonatal period, as well as specifically explore the molecular events associated with the development of CMM. There is a critical need for more non-invasive studies focusing on explaining the specific optical properties of infant skin and differentiating them from those in toddlers, older children, adolescents, and adults. We also not only need to better understand the factors influencing vitamin D synthesis in the skin but will require substantially more investigation to clarify whether the higher levels of calcitriol produced in response to UVR by infant skin specifically modulate the function of dendritic cells or repair UVB-induced DNA damage associated with skin cancer risk. In addition, future efforts should be made to refine current understanding of UVB-related immunosuppression in human infants, elucidate the time course of pigmentation in sun-exposed areas, and assess the efficacy of sun protection practices in preventing some of these changes. Furthermore, substantial work remains to be done to better define the relationship between UVR and melanogenesis in early life. Particularly important will be to elucidate the precise mechanism underlying the heightened sensitivity to UVR of neonatal mouse melanocytes, as well as efforts to establish what proportion of the differences in melanogenesis observed in human infants during the first year of life are due to sun exposure as opposed to natural developmental changes.

Future studies addressing the biologic effects of UVR on infant skin will almost certainly build on efforts already underway with transgenic mouse models to identify gene loci regulating tumor suppression, apoptosis, and cell senescence. Additional work will be needed, however, to determine factors that might predispose neonatal cells to neoplastic determination, including a lack of complete differentiation, increased numbers of melanocytes in the dermis and at the dermal/epidermal junction, and/or differences in melanocytic growth factors. In addition, efforts to extend these findings to humans will be critical, as will be efforts to determine the precise initiating events in the development of melanoma in both nevus-prone individuals and in those exposed to burning doses of UVB during early life. At the same time, future efforts should be made to determine: a) the innate characteristics of neonatal melanocytes that appear to make them particularly sensitive to UVR-induced proliferation and transformation, b) which keratinocyte to melanocyte signaling pathways might be involved in inducing migration after exposure to UVR, and c) whether there might be a specific developmental window in which these effects are most pronounced. Such efforts will be key to providing potential targets for early disease diagnosis and intervention in the development of photocarcinogenesis and other UVR-related damage traceable to exposure in the first years of life.

REFERENCES

[1]   Mancini, AJ; Lawley, L. Structure and Function of Newborn Skin. In: Eichenfield LFF, Ilona J; Esterly, Nancy B, editor. *Neonatal Dermatology*. 2nd ed. Philadelphia: Saunders Elsevier; 2008.

[2]   Nikolovski, J; Stamatas, GN; Kollias, N; Wiegand, BC. Barrier function and water-holding and transport properties of infant stratum corneum are different from adult and continue to develop through the first year of life. *J. Invest. Dermatol.* 2008, 128(7), 1728-36.

[3]   Stamatas, GN; Nikolovski, J; Luedtke, MA; Kollias, N; Wiegand, BC. Infant Skin Microstructure Assessed In Vivo Differs from Adult Skin in Organization and at the Cellular Level. *Pediatr. Dermatol.* 2009 Oct 4. [Epub ahead of print].

[4]   Vitellaro-Zuccarello, L; Cappelletti, S; Dal Pozzo Rossi, V; Sari-Gorla, M. Stereological analysis of collagen and elastic fibers in the normal human dermis: variability with age, sex, and body region. *Anat. Rec.* 1994, 238(2), 153-162.

[5]   Geller, AC; Colditz, G; Oliveria, S; Emmons, K; Jorgensen, C; Aweh, GN; et al. Use of sunscreen, sunburning rates, and tanning bed use among more than 10 000 US children and adolescents. *Pediatrics.* 2002, 109(6), 1009-14.

[6]   Dadlani, C; Orlow, SJ. Planning for a brighter future: a review of sun protection and barriers to behavioral change in children and adolescents. *Dermatol. Online J.* 2008, 14(9), 1.

[7]   Harrison, SL; Saunders, V; Nowak, M. Baseline survey of sun-protection knowledge, practices and policy in early childhood settings in Queensland, Australia. *Health Educ. Res.* 2007, 22(2), 261-71.

[8]   Thieden, E; Philipsen, PA; Sandby-Moller, J; Wulf, HC. Sunscreen use related to UV exposure, age, sex, and occupation based on personal dosimeter readings and sun-exposure behavior diaries. *Arch. Dermatol.* 2005, 141(8), 967-73.

[9]   Boldeman, C; Dal, H; Wester, U. Swedish pre-school children's UVR exposure - a comparison between two outdoor environments. *Photodermatol. Photoimmunol. Photomed* 2004, 20(1), 2-8.

[10]   Cokkinides, V; Weinstock, M; Glanz, K; Albano, J; Ward, E; Thun, M. Trends in sunburns, sun protection practices, and attitudes toward sun exposure protection and tanning among US adolescents, 1998-2004. *Pediatrics.* 2006, 118(3), 853-64.

[11]   Robinson, JK; Rademaker, AW; Sylvester, JA; Cook, B. Summer sun exposure: knowledge, attitudes, and behaviors of Midwest adolescents. *Prev. Med* .1997, 26(3), 364-72.

[12]   Davis, KJ; Cokkinides, VE; Weinstock, MA; O'Connell, MC; Wingo, PA. Summer sunburn and sun exposure among US youths ages 11 to 18: national prevalence and associated factors. *Pediatrics.* 2002, 110(1 Pt 1), 27-35.

[13]   Rigel, DS. Cutaneous ultraviolet exposure and its relationship to the development of skin cancer. *J. Am. Acad. Dermatol.* 2008, 58(5 Suppl 2), S129-32.

[14]   Hebert, AA. Photoprotection in children. *Adv. Dermatol.* 1993, 8, 309-24; discussion 325.

[15]   Elwood, JM; Jopson, J. Melanoma and sun exposure: an overview of published studies. *Int. J. Cancer.* 1997, 73(2), 198-203.

[16]   Purdue, MP; Freeman, LE; Anderson, WF; Tucker, MA. Recent trends in incidence of cutaneous melanoma among US Caucasian young adults. *J. Invest. Dermatol.* 2008, 128(12), 2905-8.

[17]   Stern, RS; Weinstein, MC; Baker, SG. Risk reduction for nonmelanoma skin cancer with childhood sunscreen use. *Arch. Dermatol.* 1986, 122(5), 537-45.

[18]   Cole, C. Sunscreen protection in the ultraviolet A region: how to measure the effectiveness. *Photodermatol. Photoimmunol. Photomed.* 2001, 17(1), 2-10.

[19]   Westerdahl, J; Olsson, H; Ingvar, C. At what age do sunburn episodes play a crucial role for the development of malignant melanoma. *Eur. J. Cancer.* 1994, 30A(11), 1647-54.

[20]   Whiteman, D; Green, A. Melanoma and sunburn. *Cancer Causes Control.* 1994, 5(6), 564-72.

[21] Wentzell, JM. Sunscreens: the ounce of prevention. *Am. Fam. Physician.* 1996, 53(5), 1713-33.

[22] Gallagher, RP; Hill, GB; Bajdik, CD; Coldman, AJ; Fincham, S; McLean, DI; et al. Sunlight exposure, pigmentation factors, and risk of nonmelanocytic skin cancer. II. Squamous cell carcinoma. *Arch. Dermatol.* 1995, 131(2), 164-9.

[23] Kricker, A; Armstrong, BK; English, DR; Heenan, PJ. Does intermittent sun exposure cause basal cell carcinoma? a case-control study in Western Australia. *Int. J. Cancer.* 1995, 60(4), 489-94.

[24] Balk, SJ; O'Connor, KG; Saraiya, M. Counseling parents and children on sun protection: a national survey of pediatricians. *Pediatrics.* 2004, 114(4), 1056-64.

[25] Harrison, SL; MacLennan, R; Speare, R; Wronski, I. Sun exposure and melanocytic naevi in young Australian children. *Lancet.* 1994, 344(8936), 1529-32.

[26] Armstrong, BK; Kricker, A. How much melanoma is caused by sun exposure? *Melanoma Res.* 1993, 3(6), 395-401.

[27] Green, A; Siskind, V; Hansen, ME; Hanson, L; Leech, P. Melanocytic nevi in schoolchildren in Queensland. *J. Am. Acad. Dermatol.* 1989, 20(6), 1054-60.

[28] Luther, H; Altmeyer, P; Garbe, C; Ellwanger, U; Jahn, S; Hoffmann, K; et al. Increase of melanocytic nevus counts in children during 5 years of follow-up and analysis of associated factors. *Arch. Dermatol.* 1996, 132(12), 1473-8.

[29] Glanz, K; Saraiya, M; Wechsler, H. Guidelines for school programs to prevent skin cancer. *MMWR Recomm. Rep.* 2002, 51(RR-4), 1-18.

[30] AAP Committee on Environmental Health. Ultraviolet light: a hazard to children. American Academy of Pediatrics. Committee on Environmental Health. *Pediatrics.* 1999, 104(2 Pt 1), 328-33.

[31] Australasian College of Dermatologists. A-Z of skin: baby and toddler protection. 2001. Available from: http://www.dermcoll.asn.au/public/a-z_of_skin-baby_toddler_protection.asp.

[32] Cancer Council of Australia. Sun protection and infants (0-12 months). 2005. Available from: http://www.cancer.org.au//File/Policy Publications/PSsunprotectioninfantsMAY05.pdf.

[33] World Health Organization. Sunshine and Health: How to Enjoy the Sun Safely. 2006. Available from: http://www.who.int/uv/publications/solaruvflyer2006.pdf.

[34] Jemal, A; Siegel, R; Ward, E; Hao, Y; Xu, J; Murray, T; et al. Cancer statistics, 2008. *CA Cancer J. Clin.* 2008, 58(2), 71-96.

[35] Osterlind, A; Tucker, MA; Stone, BJ; Jensen, OM. The Danish case-control study of cutaneous malignant melanoma. II. Importance of UV-light exposure. *Int. J. Cancer.* 1988, 42(3), 319-24.

[36] Holman, CD; Armstrong, BK; Heenan, PJ. Relationship of cutaneous malignant melanoma to individual sunlight-exposure habits. *J. Natl. Cancer Inst.* 1986, 76(3), 403-14.

[37] Green, A; MacLennan, R; Siskind, V. Common acquired naevi and the risk of malignant melanoma. *Int. J. Cancer.* 1985, 35(3), 297-300.

[38] MacKie, RM; Aitchison, T. Severe sunburn and subsequent risk of primary cutaneous malignant melanoma in scotland. *Br. J. Cancer.* 1982, 46(6), 955-60.

[39] Weinstock, MA; Colditz, GA; Willett, WC; Stampfer, MJ; Bronstein, BR; Mihm, MC, Jr.; et al. Nonfamilial cutaneous melanoma incidence in women associated with sun exposure before 20 years of age. *Pediatrics.* 1989, 84(2), 199-204.

[40] Paller, AS; Mancini, AJ. Hurwitz Clinical Pediatric Dermatology. 3rd ed: Elsevier Saunders; 2006.

[41] Green, A; Siskind, V; Bain, C; Alexander, J. Sunburn and malignant melanoma. *Br. J. Cancer.* 1985, 51(3), 393-7.

[42] Whiteman, DC; Watt, P; Purdie, DM; Hughes, MC; Hayward, NK; Green, AC. Melanocytic nevi, solar keratoses, and divergent pathways to cutaneous melanoma. *J. Natl. Cancer Inst.* 2003, 95(11), 806-12.

[43] Whiteman, DC; Stickley, M; Watt, P; Hughes, MC; Davis, MB; Green, AC. Anatomic site, sun exposure, and risk of cutaneous melanoma. *J. Clin. Oncol.* 2006, 24(19), 3172-7.

[44] Whiteman, DC; Whiteman, CA; Green, AC. Childhood sun exposure as a risk factor for melanoma: a systematic review of epidemiologic studies. *Cancer Causes Control.* 2001, 12(1), 69-82.

[45] Steinitz, R; Parkin, DM; Young, JL; Bieber, CA; Katz, L. Cancer incidence in Jewish migrants to Israel, 1961-1981. *IARC Sci. Publ.* 1989, (98), 1-311.

[46] Khlat, M; Vail, A; Parkin, M; Green, A. Mortality from melanoma in migrants to Australia: variation by age at arrival and duration of stay. *Am. J. Epidemiol.* 1992, 135(10), 1103-13.

[47] Pfahlberg, A; Kolmel, KF; Gefeller, O. Timing of excessive ultraviolet radiation and melanoma: epidemiology does not support the existence of

a critical period of high susceptibility to solar ultraviolet radiation-induced melanoma. *Br. J. Dermatol.* 2001, 144(3), 471-5.

[48] Holland, R; Harvey, I. Adult vs childhood susceptibility to melanoma: is there a difference? *Arch. Dermatol.* 2002, 138(9), 1234-5.

[49] Autier, P; Dore, JF. Influence of sun exposures during childhood and during adulthood on melanoma risk. EPIMEL and EORTC Melanoma Cooperative Group. European Organisation for Research and Treatment of Cancer. *Int. J. Cancer.* 1998, 77(4), 533-7.

[50] Whiteman, DC; Parsons, PG; Green, AC. p53 expression and risk factors for cutaneous melanoma: a case-control study. *Int. J. Cancer.* 1998, 77(6), 843-8.

[51] Thomas, NE; Edmiston, SN; Alexander, A; Millikan, RC; Groben, PA; Hao, H; et al. Number of nevi and early-life ambient UV exposure are associated with BRAF-mutant melanoma. *Cancer Epidemiol. Biomarkers Prev.* 2007, 16(5), 991-7.

[52] Swerdlow, AJ; English, J; MacKie, RM; O'Doherty, CJ; Hunter, JA; Clark, J; et al. Benign melanocytic naevi as a risk factor for malignant melanoma. *Br. Med. J. (Clin Res Ed)* 1986, 292(6535), 1555-9.

[53] Holly, EA; Kelly, JW; Shpall, SN; Chiu, SH. Number of melanocytic nevi as a major risk factor for malignant melanoma. *J. Am. Acad. Dermatol.* 1987, 17(3), 459-68.

[54] Grob, JJ; Gouvernet, J; Aymar, D; Mostaque, A; Romano, MH; Collet, AM; et al. Count of benign melanocytic nevi as a major indicator of risk for nonfamilial nodular and superficial spreading melanoma. *Cancer.* 1990, 66(2), 387-95.

[55] Garbe, C; Buttner, P; Weiss, J; Soyer, HP; Stocker, U; Kruger, S; et al. Risk factors for developing cutaneous melanoma and criteria for identifying persons at risk: multicenter case-control study of the Central Malignant Melanoma Registry of the German Dermatological Society. *J. Invest. Dermatol.* 1994, 102(5), 695-9.

[56] Crowson, AN; Magro, CM; Sanchez-Carpintero, I; Mihm, MC, Jr. The precursors of malignant melanoma. *Recent Results Cancer Res.* 2002, 160, 75-84.

[57] Thompson, SC; Jolley, D; Marks, R. Reduction of solar keratoses by regular sunscreen use. *N. Engl. J. Med.* 1993, 329(16), 1147-51.

[58] Gilchrest, BA; Eller, MS; Geller, AC; Yaar, M. The pathogenesis of melanoma induced by ultraviolet radiation. *N. Engl. J. Med.* 1999, 340(17), 1341-8.

[59] Ortonne, JP. Photoprotective properties of skin melanin. *Br. J. Dermatol.* 2002, 146 Suppl 61, 7-10.

[60] Yamaguchi, Y; Beer, J; Hearing, V. Human skin responses to UV radiation: pigment in the upper epidermis protects against DNA damage in the lower epidermis and facilitates apoptosis. *FASEB Journal.* 2006, 20(9), 1486-1488.

[61] Harrison, SL; MacLennan, R; Buettner, PG. Sun exposure and the incidence of melanocytic nevi in young Australian children. *Cancer Epidemiol. Biomarkers Prev.* 2008, 17(9), 2318-24.

[62] Whiteman, DC; Brown, RM; Purdie, DM; Hughes, MC. Melanocytic nevi in very young children: the role of phenotype, sun exposure, and sun protection. *J. Am. Acad. Dermatol.* 2005, 52(1), 40-7.

[63] Wiecker, TS; Luther, H; Buettner, P; Bauer, J; Garbe, C. Moderate sun exposure and nevus counts in parents are associated with development of melanocytic nevi in childhood: a risk factor study in 1,812 kindergarten children. *Cancer.* 2003, 97(3), 628-38.

[64] Bauer, J; Curtin, JA; Pinkel, D; Bastian, BC. Congenital melanocytic nevi frequently harbor NRAS mutations but no BRAF mutations. *J. Invest. Dermatol.* 2007, 127(1), 179-82.

[65] Branstrom, R; Kristjansson, S; Dal, H; Rodvall, Y. Sun exposure and sunburn among Swedish toddlers. *Eur. J. Cancer.* 2006, 42(10), 1441-7.

[66] Leiter, U; Garbe, C. Epidemiology of melanoma and nonmelanoma skin cancer--the role of sunlight. *Adv. Exp. Med. Biol.* 2008, 624, 89-103.

[67] Stanton, WR; Saleheen, HN; O'Riordan, D; Roy, CR. Environmental conditions and variation in levels of sun exposure among children in child care. *Int. J. Behav. Med.* 2003, 10(4), 285-98.

[68] Armstrong, BK; Kricker, A. The epidemiology of UV induced skin cancer. *J. Photochem. Photobiol. B.* 2001, 63(1-3), 8-18.

[69] Marks, R. Epidemiology of non-melanoma skin cancer and solar keratoses in Australia: a tale of self-immolation in Elysian fields. *Australas J. Dermatol.* 1997, 38 Suppl 1, S26-9.

[70] Marks, R; Jolley, D; Lectsas, S; Foley, P. The role of childhood exposure to sunlight in the development of solar keratoses and non-melanocytic skin cancer. *Med. J. Aust.* 1990, 152(2), 62-6.

[71] McGee, H; Scott, DK; Woods, GM. Neonatal exposure to UV-B radiation leads to a large reduction in Langerhans cell density, but by maturity, there is an enhanced ability of dendritic cells to stimulate T cells. *Immunol. Cell Biol.* 2006, 84(3), 259-66.

[72] Wolnicka-Glubisz, A; Noonan, FP. Neonatal susceptibility to UV induced cutaneous malignant melanoma in a mouse model. *Photochem. Photobiol. Sci.* 2006, 5(2), 254-60.

[73] Clydesdale, GJ; Dandie, GW; Muller, HK. Ultraviolet light induced injury: immunological and inflammatory effects. *Immunol. Cell Biol.* 2001, 79(6), 547-68.

[74] De Fabo, EC; Noonan, FP; Fears, T; Merlino, G. Ultraviolet B but not ultraviolet A radiation initiates melanoma. *Cancer Res.* 2004, 64(18), 6372-6.

[75] Recio, JA; Noonan, FP; Takayama, H; Anver, MR; Duray, P; Rush, WL; et al. Ink4a/arf deficiency promotes ultraviolet radiation-induced melanomagenesis. *Cancer Res.* 2002, 62(22), 6724-30.

[76] Norval, M. The mechanisms and consequences of ultraviolet-induced immunosuppression. *Prog. Biophys. Mol. Biol.* 2006, 92(1), 108-18.

[77] Sleijffers, A; Garssen, J; Vos, JG; Loveren, H. Ultraviolet light and resistance to infectious diseases. *J. Immunotoxicol.* 2004, 1(1), 3-14.

[78] Garssen, J; Vandebriel, RJ; van Loveren, H. Molecular aspects of UVB-induced immunosuppression. *Arch. Toxicol. Suppl.* 1997, 19, 97-109.

[79] Muller, HK; Bucana, C; Kripke, ML. Antigen presentation in the skin: modulation by u.v. radiation and chemical carcinogens. *Semin. Immunol.* 1992, 4(4), 205-15.

[80] Kripke, ML; Cox, PA; Alas, LG; Yarosh, DB. Pyrimidine dimers in DNA initiate systemic immunosuppression in UV-irradiated mice. *Proc. Natl. Acad. Sci. U. S. A.* 1992, 89(16), 7516-20.

[81] Godar, DE. UV doses of American children and adolescents. *Photochem. Photobiol.* 2001, 74(6), 787-93.

[82] Stanton, WR; Chakma, B; O'Riordan, DL; Eyeson-Annan, M. Sun exposure and primary prevention of skin cancer for infants and young children during autumn/winter. *Aust. N. Z. J. Public Health.* 2000, 24(2), 178-84.

[83] Moise, AF; Gies, HP; Harrison, SL. Estimation of the annual solar UVR exposure dose of infants and small children in tropical Queensland, Australia. *Photochem. Photobiol.* 1999, 69(4), 457-63.

[84] Liu, SC; Parsons, CS; Hanawalt, PC. DNA repair response in human epidermal keratinocytes from donors of different age. *J. Invest. Dermatol.* 1982, 79(5), 330-5.

[85] Liu, SC; Parsons, S; Hanawalt, PC. DNA repair in cultured keratinocytes. *J. Invest. Dermatol.* 1983, 81(1 Suppl), 179s-83s.

[86] Garmyn, M; Yaar, M; Boileau, N; Backendorf, C; Gilchrest, BA. Effect of aging and habitual sun exposure on the genetic response of cultured human keratinocytes to solar-simulated irradiation. *J. Invest. Dermatol.* 1992, 99(6), 743-8.

[87] Takahashi, Y; Moriwaki, S; Sugiyama, Y; Endo, Y; Yamazaki, K; Mori, T; et al. Decreased gene expression responsible for post-ultraviolet DNA repair synthesis in aging: a possible mechanism of age-related reduction in DNA repair capacity. *J. Invest. Dermatol.* 2005, 124(2), 435-42.

[88] Muller, HK; Malley, RC; McGee, HM; Scott, DK; Wozniak, T; Woods, GM. Effect of UV radiation on the neonatal skin immune system-implications for melanoma. *Photochem. Photobiol.* 2008, 84(1), 47-54.

[89] Kaplan, DH; Jenison, MC; Saeland, S; Shlomchik, WD; Shlomchik, MJ. Epidermal langerhans cell-deficient mice develop enhanced contact hypersensitivity. *Immunity.* 2005, 23(6), 611-20.

[90] Dewar, AL; Doherty, KV; Woods, GM; Lyons, AB; Muller, HK. Acquisition of immune function during the development of the Langerhans cell network in neonatal mice. *Immunology.* 2001, 103(1), 61-9.

[91] Simpson, CC; Woods, GM; Muller, HK. Impaired CD40-signalling in Langerhans' cells from murine neonatal draining lymph nodes: implications for neonatally induced cutaneous tolerance. *Clin. Exp. Immunol.* 2003, 132(2), 201-8.

[92] Bellette, BM; Woods, GM; Wozniak, T; Doherty, KV; Muller, HK. DEC-205lo Langerinlo neonatal Langerhans' cells preferentially utilize a wortmannin-sensitive, fluid-phase pathway to internalize exogenous antigen. *Immunology.*2003, 110(4), 466-73.

[93] Moon, EY; Noh, YW; Han, YH; Kim, SU; Kim, JM; Yu, DY; et al. T lymphocytes and dendritic cells are activated by the deletion of peroxiredoxin II (Prx II) gene. *Immunol. Lett.* 2006, 102(2), 184-90.

[94] Lehmann, B. The vitamin D3 pathway in human skin and its role for regulation of biological processes. *Photochem. Photobiol.* 2005, 81(6), 1246-51.

[95] Lehmann, B; Meurer, M. Extrarenal sites of calcitriol synthesis: the particular role of the skin. *Recent Results Cancer Res.* 2003, 164, 135-45.

[96] Lehmann, B; Sauter, W; Knuschke, P; Dressler, S; Meurer, M. Demonstration of UVB-induced synthesis of 1 alpha,25-dihydroxyvitamin D3 (calcitriol) in human skin by microdialysis. *Arch. Dermatol. Res.* 2003, 295(1), 24-8.

[97] Wagner, CL; Greer, FR. Prevention of rickets and vitamin D deficiency in infants, children, and adolescents. *Pediatrics.* 2008, 122(5), 1142-52.

[98] Reichrath, J. The challenge resulting from positive and negative effects of sunlight: how much solar UV exposure is appropriate to balance between risks of vitamin D deficiency and skin cancer? *Prog. Biophys. Mol. Biol.* 2006, 92(1), 9-16.

[99] Poduje, S; Sjerobabski-Masnec, I; Ozanic-Bulic, S. Vitamin D--the true and the false about vitamin D. *Coll. Antropol.* 2008, 32 Suppl 2, 159-62.

[100] Meindl, S; Rot, A; Hoetzenecker, W; Kato, S; Cross, HS; Elbe-Burger, A. Vitamin D receptor ablation alters skin architecture and homeostasis of dendritic epidermal T cells. *Br. J. Dermatol.* 2005, 152(2), 231-41.

[101] Lehmann, B; Knuschke, P; Meurer, M. UVB-induced conversion of 7-dehydrocholesterol to 1 alpha,25-dihydroxyvitamin D3 (calcitriol) in the human keratinocyte line HaCaT. *Photochem. Photobiol.* 2000, 72(6), 803-9.

[102] Hanneman, KK; Cooper, KD; Baron, ED. Ultraviolet immunosuppression: mechanisms and consequences. *Dermatol. Clin.* 2006, 24(1), 19-25.

[103] Guo, Z; Okamoto, H; Danno, K; Imamura, S. The effects of non-interval PUVA treatment on Langerhans cells and contact hypersensitivity. *J. Dermatol. Sci.* 1992, 3(2), 91-6.

[104] Fujita, H; Asahina, A; Komine, M; Tamaki, K. The direct action of 1alpha,25(OH)2-vitamin D3 on purified mouse Langerhans cells. *Cell Immunol.* 2007, 245(2), 70-9.

[105] Kowitz, A; Greiner, M; Thieroff-Ekerdt, R. Inhibitory effect of 1alpha,25-dihydroxyvitamin D3 on allogeneic lymphocyte stimulation and Langerhans cell maturation. *Arch. Dermatol. Res.* 1998, 290(10), 540-6.

[106] Wong, G; Gupta, R; Dixon, KM; Deo, SS; Choong, SM; Halliday, GM; et al. 1,25-Dihydroxyvitamin D and three low-calcemic analogs decrease UV-induced DNA damage via the rapid response pathway. *J. Steroid Biochem. Mol. Biol.* 2004, 89-90(1-5), 567-70.

[107] Woods, GM; Malley, RC; Muller, HK. The skin immune system and the challenge of tumour immunosurveillance. *Eur. J. Dermatol.* 2005, 15(2), 63-9.

[108] Noonan, FP; Recio, JA; Takayama, H; Duray, P; Anver, MR; Rush, WL; et al. Neonatal sunburn and melanoma in mice. *Nature.* 2001, 413(6853), 271-2.

[109] McLoone, P; Woods, GM; Norval, M. Decrease in langerhans cells and increase in lymph node dendritic cells following chronic exposure of mice to suberythemal doses of solar simulated radiation. *Photochem. Photobiol.* 2005, 81(5), 1168-73.

[110] Quelle, DE; Zindy, F; Ashmun, RA; Sherr, CJ. Alternative reading frames of the INK4a tumor suppressor gene encode two unrelated proteins capable of inducing cell cycle arrest. *Cell.* 1995, 83(6), 993-1000.

[111] Chin, L; Pomerantz, J; DePinho, RA. The INK4a/ARF tumor suppressor: one gene--two products--two pathways. *Trends Biochem. Sci.* 1998, 23(8), 291-6.

[112] Chin, L; Merlino, G; DePinho, RA. Malignant melanoma: modern black plague and genetic black box. *Genes Dev.* 1998, 12(22), 3467-81.

[113] Kannan, K; Sharpless, NE; Xu, J; O'Hagan, RC; Bosenberg, M; Chin, L. Components of the Rb pathway are critical targets of UV mutagenesis in a murine melanoma model. *Proc. Natl. Acad. Sci. U. S. A.* 2003, 100(3), 1221-5.

[114] Hacker, E; Irwin, N; Muller, HK; Powell, MB; Kay, G; Hayward, N; et al. Neonatal ultraviolet radiation exposure is critical for malignant melanoma induction in pigmented Tpras transgenic mice. *J. Invest. Dermatol.* 2005, 125(5), 1074-7.

[115] Hacker, E; Muller, HK; Irwin, N; Gabrielli, B; Lincoln, D; Pavey, S; et al. Spontaneous and UV radiation-induced multiple metastatic melanomas in Cdk4R24C/R24C/TPras mice. *Cancer Res.* 2006, 66(6), 2946-52.

[116] Walker, GJ; Kimlin, MG; Hacker, E; Ravishankar, S; Muller, HK; Beermann, F; et al. Murine neonatal melanocytes exhibit a heightened proliferative response to ultraviolet radiation and migrate to the epidermal basal layer. *J. Invest. Dermatol.* 2009, 129(1), 184-93.

[117] Abdel-Malek, ZA; Knittel, J; Kadekaro, AL; Swope, VB; Starner, R. The melanocortin 1 receptor and the UV response of human melanocytes--a shift in paradigm. *Photochem. Photobiol.* 2008, 84(2), 501-8.

[118] Jimbow, K; Uesugi, T. New melanogenesis and photobiological processes in activation and proliferation of precursor melanocytes after UV-exposure: ultrastructural differentiation of precursor melanocytes from Langerhans cells. *J. Invest. Dermatol.* 1982, 78(2), 108-15.

[119] Noonan, FP; Otsuka, T; Bang, S; Anver, MR; Merlino, G. Accelerated ultraviolet radiation-induced carcinogenesis in hepatocyte growth factor/scatter factor transgenic mice. *Cancer Res.* 2000, 60(14), 3738-43.

[120] van Schanke, A; Jongsma, MJ; Bisschop, R; van Venrooij, GM; Rebel, H; de Gruijl, FR. Single UVB overexposure stimulates melanocyte proliferation in murine skin, in contrast to fractionated or UVA-1 exposure. *J. Invest. Dermatol.* 2005, 124(1), 241-7.

[121] Silvers, WK; Mintz, B. Differences in latency and inducibility of mouse skin melanomas depending on the age and anatomic site of the skin. *Cancer Res.* 1998, 58(4), 630-2.

[122] Rivers, JK. Is there more than one road to melanoma? *Lancet.* 2004, 363(9410), 728-30.

[123] Lin, JY; Fisher, DE. Melanocyte biology and skin pigmentation. *Nature.* 2007, 445(7130), 843-50.

[124] Dixon, KM; Deo, SS; Wong, G; Slater, M; Norman, AW; Bishop, JE; et al. Skin cancer prevention: a possible role of 1,25dihydroxyvitamin D3 and its analogs. *J. Steroid Biochem. Mol. Biol.* 2005, 97(1-2), 137-43.

[125] Karasawa, M; Hosoi, J; Hashiba, H; Nose, K; Tohyama, C; Abe, E; et al. Regulation of metallothionein gene expression by 1 alpha,25-dihydroxyvitamin D3 in cultured cells and in mice. *Proc. Natl. Acad. Sci. U. S. A.* 1987, 84(24), 8810-3.

[126] Wang, WH; Li, LF; Zhang, BX; Lu, XY. Metallothionein-null mice exhibit reduced tolerance to ultraviolet B injury in vivo. *Clin. Exp. Dermatol.* 2004, 29(1), 57-61.

[127] MacLaughlin, J; Holick, MF. Aging decreases the capacity of human skin to produce vitamin D3. *J. Clin. Invest.* 1985, 76(4), 1536-8.

[128] Harpin, VA; Rutter, N. Barrier properties of the newborn infant's skin. *J. Pediatr.* 1983, 102(3), 419-25.

[129] Kalia, YN; Nonato, LB; Lund, CH; Guy, RH. Development of skin barrier function in premature infants. *J. Invest. Dermatol.* 1998, 111(2), 320-6.

[130] Yosipovitch, G; Maayan-Metzger, A; Merlob, P; Sirota, L. Skin barrier properties in different body areas in neonates. *Pediatrics.* 2000, 106(1 Pt 1), 105-8.

[131] Rutter, N; Hull, D. Water loss from the skin of term and preterm babies. *Arch. Dis. Child.* 1979, 54(11), 858-68.

[132] Visscher, MO; Chatterjee, R; Munson, KA; Pickens, WL; Hoath, SB. Changes in diapered and nondiapered infant skin over the first month of life. *Pediatr. Dermatol.* 2000, 17(1), 45-51.

[133] Hoeger, PH; Enzmann, CC. Skin physiology of the neonate and young infant: a prospective study of functional skin parameters during early infancy. *Pediatr. Dermatol.* 2002, 19(3), 256-62.

[134] Menon, GK. New insights into skin structure: scratching the surface. *Adv. Drug Deliv. Rev.* 2002, 54 Suppl 1, S3-17.

[135] Hoath, SB. The stickiness of newborn skin: bioadhesion and the epidermal barrier. *J. Pediatr.* 1997, 131(3), 338-40.

[136] McLoone, P; Simics, E; Barton, A; Norval, M; Gibbs, N. An action spectrum for the production of cis-urocanic acid in human skin in vivo. *Journal of Investigative Dermatology* 2005, 124, 1071-1074.

[137] Behne, MJ; Barry, NP; Hanson, KM; Aronchik, I; Clegg, RW; Gratton, E; et al. Neonatal development of the stratum corneum pH gradient: localization and mechanisms leading to emergence of optimal barrier function. *J. Invest. Dermatol.* 2003, 120(6), 998-1006.

[138] Lock-Andersen, J; Knudstorp, ND; Wulf, HC. Facultative skin pigmentation in caucasians: an objective biological indicator of lifetime exposure to ultraviolet radiation? *Br. J. Dermatol.* 1998, 138(5), 826-32.

[139] Agren, J; Sjors, G; Sedin, G. Ambient humidity influences the rate of skin barrier maturation in extremely preterm infants. *J. Pediatr.* 2006, 148(5), 613-7.

[140] Chiou, YB; Blume-Peytavi, U. Stratum corneum maturation. A review of neonatal skin function. *Skin. Pharmacol. Physiol.* 2004, 17(2), 57-66.

[141] Giusti, F; Martella, A; Bertoni, L; Seidenari, S. Skin barrier, hydration, and pH of the skin of infants under 2 years of age. *Pediatr. Dermatol.* 2001, 18(2), 93-6.

[142] Quaglino, D, Jr.; Bergamini, G; Boraldi, F; Pasquali Ronchetti, I. Ultrastructural and morphometrical evaluations on normal human dermal connective tissue--the influence of age, sex and body region. *Br. J. Dermatol.* 1996, 134(6), 1013-22.

[143] Kikuchi, K; Kobayashi, H; O'Goshi, K; Tagami, H. Impairment of skin barrier function is not inherent in atopic dermatitis patients: a prospective study conducted in newborns. *Pediatr. Dermatol.* 2006, 23(2), 109-13.

[144] Saijo, S; Tagami, H. Dry skin of newborn infants: functional analysis of the stratum corneum. *Pediatr. Dermatol.* 1991, 8(2), 155-9.

[145] Lund, CH; Nonato, LB; Kuller, JM; Franck, LS; Cullander, C; Durand, DJ. Disruption of barrier function in neonatal skin associated with adhesive removal. *J. Pediatr.* 1997, 131(3), 367-72.

[146] Rawlings, AV; Scott, IR; Harding, CR; Bowser, PA. Stratum corneum moisturization at the molecular level. *J. Invest. Dermatol.* 1994, 103(5), 731-41.

[147] Pierard, GE; Goffin, V; Hermanns-Le, T; Pierard-Franchimont, C. Corneocyte desquamation. *Int. J. Mol. Med.* 2000, 6(2), 217-21.

[148] Sato, J; Yanai, M; Hirao, T; Denda, M. Water content and thickness of the stratum corneum contribute to skin surface morphology. *Arch. Dermatol. Res.* 2000, 292(8), 412-7.

[149] Bouwstra, JA; Honeywell-Nguyen, PL; Gooris, GS; Ponec, M. Structure of the skin barrier and its modulation by vesicular formulations. *Prog. Lipid Res.* 2003, 42(1), 1-36.

[150] Fluhr, JW; Mao-Qiang, M; Brown, BE; Hachem, JP; Moskowitz, DG; Demerjian, M; et al. Functional consequences of a neutral pH in neonatal rat stratum corneum. *J. Invest. Dermatol.* 2004, 123(1), 140-51.

[151] Rawlings, AV; Matts, PJ. Stratum corneum moisturization at the molecular level: an update in relation to the dry skin cycle. *J. Invest. Dermatol.* 2005, 124(6), 1099-110.

[152] Mack, MC; Tierney, N; Ruvolo, E; Stamatas, GN; Martin, K; Kollias, N. Development of solar UVR-related pigmentation begins as early as the first summer of life. *J. Invest. Dermatol. (in press)* 2010.

[153] Grande, R; Gutierrez, E; Latorre, E; Arguelles, F. Physiological variations in the pigmentation of newborn infants. *Hum. Biol.* 1994, 66(3), 495-507.

[154] Park, JH; Lee, MH. A study of skin color by melanin index according to site, gestational age, birth weight and season of birth in Korean neonates. *J. Korean Med. Sci.* 2005, 20(1), 105-8.

[155] Watanabe, M; Ohki, Y; Yoshizawa, Y; Inoue, Y; Tokuyama, K; Morikawa, A. Maturational changes in skin color of Japanese newborn infants. *Neonatology.* 2007, 91(4), 275-80.

[156] Gilchrest, BA; Eller, MS. DNA photodamage stimulates melanogenesis and other photoprotective responses. *J. Investig. Dermatol. Symp. Proc.* 1999, 4(1), 35-40.

[157] Moore, C; Murphy, MM; Keast, DR; Holick, MF. Vitamin D intake in the United States. *J. Am. Diet. Assoc.* 2004, 104(6), 980-3.

[158] Rajakumar, K; Thomas, SB. Reemerging nutritional rickets: a historical perspective. *Arch. Pediatr. Adolesc. Med.* 2005, 159(4), 335-41.

[159] Pettifor, JM. Rickets and vitamin D deficiency in children and adolescents. *Endocrinol. Metab. Clin. North Am.* 2005, 34(3), 537-53, vii.

[160] Nesby-O'Dell, S; Scanlon, KS; Cogswell, ME; Gillespie, C; Hollis, BW; Looker, AC; et al. Hypovitaminosis D prevalence and determinants among African American and white women of reproductive age: third National Health and Nutrition Examination Survey, 1988-1994. *Am. J. Clin. Nutr.* 2002, 76(1), 187-92.

[161] Scanlon, KS. Vitamin D expert panel meeting, October 11-12, Atlanta, Georgia: final report. 2001. Available from: www.cdc.gov/nccdphp/ dnpa/ nutrition/pdf/Vitamin_D_Expert_Panel_Meeting.pdf <http://www. cdc.gov/nccdphp/dnpa/nutrition/pdf/Vitamin_D_Expert_Panel_Meeting. pdf>.

[162] Looker, AC; Dawson-Hughes, B; Calvo, MS; Gunter, EW; Sahyoun, NR. Serum 25-hydroxyvitamin D status of adolescents and adults in two seasonal subpopulations from NHANES III. *Bone.* 2002, 30(5), 771-7.

[163] Harkness, LS; Bonny, AE. Calcium and vitamin D status in the adolescent: key roles for bone, body weight, glucose tolerance, and estrogen biosynthesis. *J. Pediatr. Adolesc. Gynecol.* 2005, 18(5), 305-11.

[164] Harkness, LS; Cromer, BA. Vitamin D deficiency in adolescent females. *J. Adolesc. Health.* 2005, 37(1), 75.

[165] Cheng, S; Tylavsky, F; Kroger, H; Karkkainen, M; Lyytikainen, A; Koistinen, A; et al. Association of low 25-hydroxyvitamin D concentrations with elevated parathyroid hormone concentrations and low cortical bone density in early pubertal and prepubertal Finnish girls. *Am. J. Clin. Nutr.* 2003, 78(3), 485-92.

[166] Tylavsky, FA; Ryder, KA; Lyytikainen, A; Cheng, S. Vitamin D, parathyroid hormone, and bone mass in adolescents. *J. Nutr.* 2005, 135(11), 2735S-8S.

[167] DeBar, LL; Ritenbaugh, C; Aickin, M; Orwoll, E; Elliot, D; Dickerson, J; et al. Youth: a health plan-based lifestyle intervention increases bone mineral density in adolescent girls. *Arch. Pediatr. Adolesc. Med.* 2006, 160(12), 1269-76.

[168] El-Hajj Fuleihan, G; Nabulsi, M; Choucair, M; Salamoun, M; Hajj Shahine, C; Kizirian, A; et al. Hypovitaminosis D in healthy schoolchildren. *Pediatrics.* 2001, 107(4), E53.

[169] Marwaha, RK; Tandon, N; Reddy, DR; Aggarwal, R; Singh, R; Sawhney, RC; et al. Vitamin D and bone mineral density status of healthy schoolchildren in northern India. *Am. J. Clin. Nutr.* 2005, 82(2), 477-82.

[170] Lapatsanis, D; Moulas, A; Cholevas, V; Soukakos, P; Papadopoulou, ZL; Challa, A. Vitamin D: a necessity for children and adolescents in Greece. *Calcif. Tissue Int.* 2005, 77(6), 348-55.

[171] Hill, TR; Flynn, A; Kiely, M; Cashman, KD. Prevalence of suboptimal vitamin D status in young, adult and elderly Irish subjects. *Ir. Med. J.* 2006, 99(2), 48-9.

[172] Primary vitamin D deficiency in children. *Drug Ther. Bull.* 2006, 44(2), 12-6.

[173] Gordon, CM; Feldman, HA; Sinclair, L; Williams, AL; Kleinman, PK; Perez-Rossello, J; et al. Prevalence of vitamin D deficiency among healthy infants and toddlers. *Arch. Pediatr. Adolesc. Med.* 2008, 162(6), 505-12.

[174] Grant, WB; Garland, CF; Holick, MF. Comparisons of estimated economic burdens due to insufficient solar ultraviolet irradiance and vitamin D and excess solar UV irradiance for the United States. *Photochem. Photobiol.* 2005, 81(6), 1276-86.

[175] Wolpowitz, D; Gilchrest, BA. The vitamin D questions: how much do you need and how should you get it? *J. Am. Acad. Dermatol.* 2006, 54(2), 301-17.

[176] Lucas, RM; Ponsonby, AL. Considering the potential benefits as well as adverse effects of sun exposure: can all the potential benefits be provided by oral vitamin D supplementation? *Prog. Biophys. Mol. Biol.* 2006, 92(1), 140-9.

[177] Matsuoka, LY; Wortsman, J; Dannenberg, MJ; Hollis, BW; Lu, Z; Holick, MF. Clothing prevents ultraviolet-B radiation-dependent photosynthesis of vitamin D3. *J. Clin. Endocrinol. Metab.* 1992, 75(4), 1099-103.

[178] Matsuoka, LY; Wortsman, J; Haddad, JG; Kolm, P; Hollis, BW. Racial pigmentation and the cutaneous synthesis of vitamin D. *Arch. Dermatol.* 1991, 127(4), 536-8.

[179] Matsuoka, LY; Wortsman, J; Hollis, BW. Suntanning and cutaneous synthesis of vitamin D3. *J. Lab. Clin. Med.* 1990, 116(1), 87-90.

[180] Matsuoka, LY; Wortsman, J; Hollis, BW. Use of topical sunscreen for the evaluation of regional synthesis of vitamin D3. *J. Am. Acad. Dermatol.* 1990, 22(5 Pt 1), 772-5.

[181] Binkley, N; Novotny, R; Krueger, D; Kawahara, T; Daida, YG; Lensmeyer, G; et al. Low vitamin D status despite abundant sun exposure. *J. Clin. Endocrinol. Metab.* 2007, 92(6), 2130-5.

[182] Maisels, MJ; Watchko, JF. Treatment of jaundice in low birthweight infants. *Arch. Dis. Child Fetal Neonatal. Ed.* 2003, 88(6), F459-63.

[183] Maisels, MJ; McDonagh, AF. Phototherapy for neonatal jaundice. *N. Engl. J. Med.* 2008, 358(9), 920-8.

[184] McDonagh, AF. Sunlight-induced mutation of bilirubin in a long-distance runner. *N. Engl. J. Med.* 1986, 314(2), 121-2.

[185] McDonagh, AF. Ex uno plures: the concealed complexity of bilirubin species in neonatal blood samples. *Pediatrics.* 2006, 118(3), 1185-7.

[186] Myara, A; Sender, A; Valette, V; Rostoker, C; Paumier, D; Capoulade, C; et al. Early changes in cutaneous bilirubin and serum bilirubin isomers during intensive phototherapy of jaundiced neonates with blue and green light. *Biol. Neonate.* 1997, 71(2), 75-82.

[187] Kopelman, AE; Brown, RS; Odell, GB. The "bronze" baby syndrome: a complication of phototherapy. *J. Pediatr.* 1972, 81(3), 466-72.

[188] Rubaltelli, FF; Jori, G; Reddi, E. Bronze baby syndrome: a new porphyrin-related disorder. *Pediatr. Res.* 1983, 17(5), 327-30.

[189] Onishi, S; Itoh, S; Isobe, K; Togari, H; Kitoh, H; Nishimura, Y. Mechanism of development of bronze baby syndrome in neonates treated with phototherapy. *Pediatrics.* 1982, 69(3), 273-6.

[190] Ashley, JR; Littler, CM; Burgdorf, WH; Brann, BSt. Bronze baby syndrome. Report of a case. *J. Am. Acad. Dermatol.* 1985, 12(2 Pt 1), 325-8.

[191] Purcell, SM; Wians, FH, Jr.; Ackerman, NB, Jr.; Davis, BM. Hyperbiliverdinemia in the bronze baby syndrome. *J. Am. Acad. Dermatol.* 1987, 16(1 Pt 2), 172-7.

[192] Kearns, GL; Williams, BJ; Timmons, OD. Fluorescein phototoxicity in a premature infant. *J. Pediatr.* 1985, 107(5), 796-8.

[193] Burry, JN; Lawrence, JR. Phototoxic blisters from high frusemide dosage. *Br. J. Dermatol.* 1976, 94(5), 495-9.

[194] Porat, R; Gilbert, S; Magilner, D. Methylene blue-induced phototoxicity: an unrecognized complication. *Pediatrics.* 1996, 97(5), 717-21.

[195] Mallon, E; Wojnarowska, F; Hope, P; Elder, G. Neonatal bullous eruption as a result of transient porphyrinemia in a premature infant with hemolytic disease of the newborn. *J. Am. Acad. Dermatol.* 1995, 33(2 Pt 2), 333-6.

[196] Paller, AS; Eramo, LR; Farrell, EE; Millard, DD; Honig, PJ; Cunningham, BB. Purpuric phototherapy-induced eruption in transfused neonates: relation to transient porphyrinemia. *Pediatrics.* 1997, 100(3 Pt 1), 360-4.

[197] Tonz, O; Vogt, J; Filippini, L; Simmler, F; Wachsmuth, ED; Winterhalter, KH. [Severe light dermatosis following photo therapy in a newborn infant with congenital erythropoietic urophyria]. *Helv. Paediatr. Acta.* 1975, 30(1), 47-56.

[198] Valaes, T; Petmezaki, S; Henschke, C; Drummond, GS; Kappas, A. Control of jaundice in preterm newborns by an inhibitor of bilirubin production: studies with tin-mesoporphyrin. *Pediatrics.* 1994, 93(1), 1-11.

[199] Dollberg, S; Atherton, HD; Hoath, SB. Effect of different phototherapy lights on incubator characteristics and dynamics under three modes of servocontrol. *Am. J. Perinatol.* 1995, 12(1), 55-60.

[200] Maayan-Metzger, A; Yosipovitch, G; Hadad, E; Sirota, L. Transepidermal water loss and skin hydration in preterm infants during phototherapy. *Am. J. Perinatol.* 2001, 18(7), 393-6.

[201] Csoma, Z; Hencz, P; Orvos, H; Kemeny, L; Dobozy, A; Dosa-Racz, E; et al. Neonatal blue-light phototherapy could increase the risk of dysplastic nevus development. *Pediatrics.* 2007, 119(6), 1269.

[202] Matichard, E; Le Henanff, A; Sanders, A; Leguyadec, J; Crickx, B; Descamps, V. Effect of neonatal phototherapy on melanocytic nevus count in children. *Arch. Dermatol.* 2006, 142(12), 1599-604.

[203] Bauer, J; Buttner, P; Luther, H; Wiecker, TS; Mohrle, M; Garbe, C. Blue light phototherapy of neonatal jaundice does not increase the risk for melanocytic nevus development. *Arch. Dermatol.* 2004, 140(4), 493-4.

[204] Mahe, E; Beauchet, A; Aegerter, P; Saiag, P. Neonatal blue-light phototherapy does not increase nevus count in 9-year-old children. *Pediatrics.* 2009, 123(5), e896-900.

INDEX

A

absorption, 3, 4, 20
acid, 1, 20, 42
actinic keratosis, 11
activation, 18, 40
acute, 7, 10, 17
adolescence, 11
adolescent behavior, 9
adolescent female, 44
adolescents, 4, 27, 29, 31, 32, 37, 39, 43, 44, 45
adult, 4, 5, 9, 13, 14, 15, 16, 19, 20, 21, 22, 31, 45
adulthood, 5, 9, 12, 16, 18, 35
adults, 4, 5, 8, 12, 18, 21, 22, 23, 26, 29, 32, 44
African American, 44
age, vii, 7, 8, 9, 10, 11, 14, 15, 21, 23, 25, 27, 31, 32, 34, 37, 38, 41, 42, 43, 44
agents, 14, 16, 20, 26
aging, vii, 4, 7, 14, 38
aging process, 7
air, 23
allogeneic, 16, 39
alternative hypothesis, 17
alters, 16, 17, 39
American Academy of Pediatrics (AAP), 1, 23, 33

animal models, vii, 5, 13, 17, 19, 29
animal studies, 16
animals, 18
antigen, 14, 17, 38
antigen-presenting cell, 14
antioxidant, 19
anti-tumor, 18
apoptosis, 16, 18, 19, 30, 36
ARF, 40
atopic dermatitis, 21, 42
attitudes, 32
avoidance, 7, 9, 23

B

B cells, 18
babies, 20, 41
basal cell carcinoma, 1, 7, 11, 33
basal layer, 11, 18, 40
behavior, 9, 32
behavioral change, 31
benefits, 23, 45
benign, 9, 35
bilirubin, 3, 25, 26, 46, 47
biliverdin, 26
biological processes, 38
biometry, 10

biosynthesis, 44
birth, 20, 21, 23, 25, 43
birth weight, 25, 43
blood, 25, 26, 27, 46
blood flow, 27
body mass, 23
body weight, 44
bone density, 44
bone mass, 44
broad spectrum, 23
burn, 11, 12
burning, 10, 30
buttocks, 21

C

cancer, 4, 8, 13, 33, 41
capacitance, 21
capillary, 4
carcinogenesis, 41
carcinogenic, 17
carcinogens, 16, 37
carcinoma, 1, 7, 33
carcinomas, 11
case study, 9
Caucasian, 10, 12, 22, 32
cell, vii, 1, 3, 5, 7, 11, 13, 15, 16, 17, 18, 29,
    30, 33, 36, 38, 39, 40
cell body, 18
cell culture, vii, 5, 13, 29
cell cycle, 40
cell growth, 15
cell membranes, 3
chemical agents, 18
chemokines, 16
childhood, 4, 7, 8, 9, 11, 12, 16, 27, 31, 32,
    35, 36
children, 4, 5, 7, 8, 9, 10, 11, 12, 13, 19, 23,
    27, 29, 31, 32, 33, 36, 37, 39, 43, 45, 47
cholestasis, 26
clinical trial, vii, 5, 13, 26
clinical trials, vii, 5, 13, 26
clinically significant, 26
cohort, 20
collagen, 3, 4, 20, 31

complexity, 46
complications, 11, 26
components, 14
compounds, 16, 19
concentration, 21, 22, 25
conjugated bilirubin, 25
conjugation, 25
connective tissue, 20, 42
control, 7, 8, 11, 27, 33, 34, 35
control group, 27
controlled trials, 26
conversion, 39
copper, 26
critical period, 9, 35
culture, vii, 5, 16, 29
cytokines, 14, 15, 16

D

death, 25
deaths, 8
deficiency, 23, 37, 44
dendrites, 15
dendritic cell, 14, 15, 17, 19, 29, 36, 38, 40
density, 10, 15, 17, 20, 21, 36, 44
deoxyribonucleic acid, 1
derivatives, 26
dermatitis, 21
dermatologists, 23
dermatosis, 47
dermis, 3, 30, 31
destruction, 3
developmental change, 30
diet, 19
differentiation, 13, 14, 15, 30, 40
diffuse reflectance, 20, 22
diffusion, 21
direct action, 19, 39
disorder, 46
distribution, 15, 20, 21
DNA, 1, 3, 9, 10, 13, 14, 18, 19, 23, 29, 36,
    37, 38, 39, 43
DNA damage, 19, 23, 29, 36, 39
DNA repair, 14, 18, 37, 38
donors, 14, 37

dosage, 46
drugs, 26
duration, 10, 21, 34

E

ears, 37
elastin, 3, 20
elderly, 45
encephalopathy, 25
endothelial cells, 14
energy, 3, 25
environment, 16, 18, 20, 27
environmental conditions, 20
epidemiologic studies, 7, 9, 34
epidemiology, 34, 36
epidermis, 4, 11, 17, 20, 22, 36
erythematous, 26
estrogen, 44
ethnicity, 10
excision, 14
exposure, vii, 3, 4, 5, 7, 8, 9, 10, 11, 12, 13,
    14, 16, 17, 18, 19, 23, 25, 26, 30, 32, 33,
    34, 35, 36, 37, 38, 39, 40, 41, 42, 45
external influences, 22
extracellular matrix, 4, 20
eyes, 8, 10, 27

F

factorial, 18
family, 8, 26
family history, 26
females, 44
fetus, 20
fibers, 3, 4, 20, 31
fibrils, 3
fibroblasts, 14
fluid, 27, 38
fluorescence, 3
focusing, 29
free radicals, 14
functional analysis, 42

G

gene, 14, 30, 38, 40, 41
gene expression, 38, 41
generation, 3, 16, 26
genes, 14
gestation, 27
gestational age, 25, 43
girls, 44
glucose, 44
glucose tolerance, 44
growth, 15, 16, 18, 30, 41
growth factor, 15, 16, 30, 41
growth factors, 15, 16, 30
guidelines, 25

H

hair follicle, 18
health, 5, 7, 44
health effects, 7
heat, 3, 25, 27
hemoglobin, 3, 4, 22
hepatocyte, 41
hepatocyte growth factor, 41
homeostasis, 39
hormone, 15, 44
human, vii, 5, 7, 12, 13, 14, 16, 18, 19, 20,
    29, 31, 37, 38, 39, 40, 41, 42
human papilloma virus, 12
humans, 17, 18, 30
humidity, 42
hydration, 4, 20, 21, 27, 42, 47
hydrophilicity, 21
hyperbilirubinemia, 25, 26
hypersensitivity, 38, 39
hypothesis, 17

I

IARC, 34
IL-1, 14, 16
immune function, 4, 38
immune reaction, 14

immune response, 14, 15, 16, 17
immune system, 1, 13, 14, 15, 17, 38, 39
immunity, 7, 18
immunological, 37
immunomodulatory, 14, 15, 16, 19
immunosuppression, 8, 12, 13, 16, 18, 19, 29, 37, 39
immunosurveillance, 39
in vitro, 15, 16
in vivo, 13, 20, 21, 22, 41, 42
incidence, vii, 32, 34, 36
induction, 18, 40
inelastic, 3
infancy, 7, 9, 12, 16, 20, 42
infants, 3, 4, 5, 7, 8, 9, 10, 13, 20, 21, 22, 23, 25, 26, 27, 29, 33, 37, 39, 42, 43, 45, 46
infection, 12, 15
infectious diseases, 37
inflammation, 7, 15
inflammatory, 16, 17, 37
inflammatory mediators, 17
inflammatory response, 17
infrared, 20
infrared spectroscopy, 20
inhibitor, 47
injury, 37, 41
instruments, 21
integrity, 22
interactions, 4
interval, 39
intervention, 30, 44
invasive, 11, 20
irradiation, 14, 38
isomers, 46

J

jaundice, vii, 5, 25, 26, 27, 29, 46, 47

K

keratin, 3
keratinocyte, 14, 19, 30, 39

keratinocytes, 10, 14, 15, 16, 18, 19, 37, 38
kernicterus, 25
kidney, 15
kindergarten, 36
kindergarten children, 36

L

Langerhans cells, 1, 14, 39, 40
latency, 41
lesions, 10, 11
lifestyle, 44
life-threatening, 11
lifetime, 8, 10, 11, 42
light emitting diode, 27
light scattering, 3, 20
limitations, 13
lipid, 21, 43
lipids, 20
liver, 15, 25
localization, 42
low birthweight, 46
lymph, 17, 18, 38, 40
lymph node, 17, 18, 38, 40
lymphatic, 14
lymphocyte, 39

M

macrophages, 14, 15
maintenance, 15
malignancy, 8
malignant, 1, 7, 8, 9, 10, 11, 18, 32, 34, 35, 37, 40
malignant melanoma, 1, 7, 8, 18, 32, 34, 35, 37, 40
mammals, 18
mast cells, 14, 15
matrix, 4, 20
maturation, 15, 16, 20, 39, 42
maturation process, 20
measurement, 13, 21
measures, 8, 23
mediators, 17

melanin, 3, 4, 5, 18, 19, 20, 22, 36, 43
Melanocytes, 18
melanogenesis, 22, 30, 40, 43
melanoma, vii, 4, 7, 8, 9, 10, 17, 18, 27, 30, 32, 33, 34, 35, 36, 37, 38, 39, 40, 41
melanosomes, 18
men, 11
Metallothionein, 41
metastasis, 11
metastasizes, 11
metastatic, 40
methylene, 26
mice, 16, 17, 18, 19, 37, 38, 39, 40, 41
microdialysis, 38
microenvironment, 13, 14, 18, 29
microscopy, 20
migrants, 8, 34
migration, 30
models, vii, 5, 13, 16, 17, 18, 19, 29, 30
modulation, 14, 15, 37, 43
molecular weight, 25
molecules, 3, 15, 19, 20
monocytes, 14
morphology, 15, 22, 43
mothers, 20, 22
mouse, 18, 19, 30, 37, 39, 41
mouse model, 18, 37
murine models, 16
mutagenesis, 40
mutant, 35
mutation, 11, 46
mutations, 9, 11, 16, 18, 19, 36

N

natural, 1, 20, 21, 30
neonatal, vii, 5, 15, 16, 17, 18, 19, 20, 21, 25, 26, 27, 29, 30, 38, 40, 42, 43, 46, 47
neonate, 42
neonates, 15, 17, 26, 41, 43, 46
neoplasm, 11
neoplasms, 9
neoplastic, 30
neuropeptides, 14
neutrophil, 17

nevus, 10, 27, 30, 33, 36, 47
nodes, 17
non-invasive, 13, 20, 22, 29
normal, 14, 20, 25, 31, 42
nuclei, 3
nursery school, 10
nutrition, 44

O

oncogene, 14
optical, 4, 29
optical properties, 4, 29
optics, 22
oral, 23, 45
organelles, 3
organism, vii
oxidation, 26
oxidative, 15
oxidative damage, 15

P

parathyroid hormone, 44
parents, 10, 33, 36
pathogenesis, 35
pathogens, 14
pathways, 34, 40
patients, 42
pediatric, 8
peers, 12
perinatal, 20
peripheral blood, 27
permeability, 17
peroxiredoxins, 15
personal history, 8
pH values, 21
phenotype, 36
photochemical, 25
photon, 3
photosynthesis, 45
physiology, 42
pigments, 26
placebo, 26

plague, 40
play, 9, 15, 16, 18, 27, 32
plurality, 3
pollution, 23
population, 8, 9, 11
porphyria, 26
porphyrins, 26
postpartum, 21
premature infant, 41, 46
preschool children, 10
preschoolers, 10
preterm infants, 27, 42, 47
prevention, 16, 33, 37, 41
primary care, 23
production, 15, 16, 18, 19, 23, 42, 47
prognosis, 8
proliferation, 13, 15, 17, 18, 30, 40, 41
propagation, 3
prophylactic, 25
prostaglandins, 14
protection, 5, 7, 20, 22, 23, 29, 31, 32, 33, 36
protective clothing, 23
protective role, 15
protein, 15
proteins, 15, 22, 40
puberty, 28
public, 5, 7, 33
public health, 5, 7
pyrimidine, 16, 19

Q

questionnaire, 10

R

radiation, vii, 1, 5, 7, 14, 17, 23, 34, 35, 36, 37, 38, 40, 41, 42, 45
Raman spectra, 21
rat, 43
recreational, 8, 11
repair, 14, 16, 18, 19, 29, 37, 38
replication, 14

reproductive age, 44
resistance, 37
resolution, 21
responsiveness, 23
retention, 17
rickets, 39, 43
risk, 4, 8, 9, 10, 11, 12, 17, 18, 19, 27, 29, 33, 34, 35, 36, 47
risk factors, 8, 11, 27, 35
risks, vii, 5, 7, 8, 13, 23, 39

S

scatter, 22, 41
scattering, 3, 4, 20
sclera, 25
senescence, 30
sensitivity, 17, 19, 30
sensitization, 26
sequelae, 26
serum, 25, 26, 46
severity, 8, 10
sex, 12, 31, 32, 42
shape, 25
signaling pathways, 30
signalling, 38
signs, 22
SIS, 1, 13, 14, 15, 16, 17, 29
skin, vii, 1, 3, 4, 5, 7, 8, 9, 10, 11, 12, 13, 14, 15, 16, 17, 18, 19, 20, 21, 22, 23, 25, 26, 27, 29, 30, 32, 33, 36, 37, 38, 39, 41, 42, 43, 47
skin cancer, 4, 8, 11, 13, 18, 19, 29, 32, 33, 36, 37, 39
skin conductance, 21
skin diseases, vii
solar, 1, 4, 5, 10, 11, 12, 13, 14, 22, 34, 35, 36, 37, 38, 39, 40, 43, 45
somatic mutations, 9
species, 46
spectroscopy, 20, 22
spectrum, 11, 23, 26, 42
SPF, 8
squamous cell carcinoma, 1, 7, 11
statistics, 5, 34

steady state, 20
Stefin A, 15
steroid, 39, 41
summer, 10, 22, 23, 43
sun, 33, 36, 37
sunlight, 8, 9, 11, 12, 23, 27, 34, 36, 39
suppression, 13, 18, 30
suppressor, 40
surface area, 5, 20, 26
survival, 15
susceptibility, 17, 18, 35, 37
syndrome, 26, 46
synthesis, 14, 23, 29, 38, 45

T

T cells, 15, 16, 18, 36, 39
T lymphocytes, 14, 15, 38
targets, 30, 40
therapy, 26, 47
threshold, 10, 23
tissue, 3, 4, 11, 15, 16, 17, 20, 26, 42
toddlers, 10, 23, 29, 36, 45
tolerance, 14, 17, 18, 38, 41, 44
toxicity, 26
transformation, 10, 18, 30
transgenic, 17, 18, 30, 40, 41
transgenic mice, 17, 18, 40, 41
transgenic mouse, 18, 30
transparent, 3
transport, 18, 31
tumor, 16, 18, 30, 39, 40
tumors, 16
turnover, 20

U

ultraviolet, vii, 1, 5, 32, 33, 34, 35, 37, 38, 39, 40, 41, 42, 45
ultraviolet B, 41
ultraviolet light, 5

unconjugated bilirubin, 25
United States, 11, 43, 45
urine, 26
UV exposure, 32, 35, 39
UV radiation, 36, 38, 40

V

vasculature, 4
virus infection, 12
visible, 20
vitamin D, 15, 16, 19, 23, 29, 38, 39, 41, 43, 44, 45
vitamin D deficiency, 23, 39, 43, 45
vitamin D receptor, 15, 16
vulnerability, 22

W

water, 1, 20, 21, 22, 27, 31, 47
water absorption, 21
water desorption, 22
wavelengths, 26
weight ratio, 5
white women, 44
winter, 37
women, 4, 34, 44
World Health Organization, 33

X

xeroderma pigmentosum, 8, 12

Y

young adults, 32
young women, 4
younger children, 27